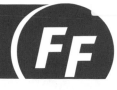

*FAST FACTS*

# Benign Prostatic

Hyperplasia

# 4 Week Loan

This book is due for return on or before the last date shown below

| | | |
|---|---|---|
| 2 2 MAR 2011 | | |
| | | |

University of Cumbria

HEALTH PRESS
Oxford

Fast Facts – Benign Prostatic Hyperplasia
First published 1995
Second edition 1997
Third edition 1999
Fourth edition September 2002
Fifth edition January 2005

Health Press Limited,
Elizabeth House, Queen Street, Abingdon,
Oxford OX14 3LN, UK
Tel: +44 (0)1235 523233
Fax: +44 (0)1235 523238

Book orders can be placed by telephone or via the website.
For regional distributors or to order via the website, please go to:
www.fastfacts.com
For telephone orders, please call 01752 202301 (UK) or
800 538 1287 (North America, toll free).

Fast Facts is a trademark of Health Press Limited.

A CIP catalogue record for this title is available from the British Library.

ISBN 1-903734-58-4

Kirby, RS (Roger)
Fast Facts – Benign Prostatic Hyperplasia/
Roger S Kirby, John D McConnell

Illustrated by Dee McLean, London, UK.
Typesetting and page layout by Zed, Oxford, UK.
Printed by Fine Print (Services) Ltd, Oxford, UK.

Printed with vegetable inks on fully biodegradable and
recyclable paper manufactured from sustainable forests.

444     001
Low emissions
during production

Low
chlorine

Sustainable
forests

# Glossary

5α-R: 5α-reductase

**5α-reductase inhibitors:** drugs that inhibit the enzyme 5α-reductase, and thus lower prostatic dihydrotestosterone levels and can result in some decrease in prostate size (e.g. dutasteride, finasteride)

$\alpha_1$-**blockers:** drugs that block $\alpha_1$-adrenoceptors in the prostate, thereby relieving outflow obstruction; examples include alfuzosin, doxazosin, indoramin, tamsulosin and terazosin

**AUR:** acute urinary retention

**BII:** BPH impact index

**Bladder outlet obstruction (outflow obstruction, BOO):** an obstruction in the bladder outlet, resulting from anatomical (e.g. BPH) or neurogenic causes

**BPE:** benign prostatic enlargement

**BPH:** benign prostatic hyperplasia

**Combination therapy:** the combination of an α-blocker with a 5α-reductase inhibitor to reduce the risk of BPH progression

**Detrusor muscle:** the smooth muscle in the bladder wall

**DHT:** dihydrotestosterone, the active metabolite of testosterone

**Diverticulum** (plural diverticula): a pouch or sac in a hollow organ, usually the bladder

**DRE:** digital rectal examination

**ED:** erectile dysfunction

**ELAP:** endoscopic laser ablation of the prostate (also called VLAP)

**Holmium laser:** a laser that permits bloodless removal of prostate tissue

**HoLRP:** holmium laser resection of the prostate

**Hyperplasia:** an increase in the number of normal cells in a tissue

**Irritative symptoms:** symptoms arising from detrusor instability, such as urgency, frequency, nocturia and urge incontinence

**IVU:** intravenous urogram

**LUTS:** lower urinary tract symptoms associated with, but not always the result of, BPH

**Microscopic BPH:** BPH that is detectable only histologically

**MTOPS:** Medical Treatment of Prostatic Symptoms study

**Nocturia:** necessity to rise from bed at night to pass urine

**Obstructive symptoms:** symptoms arising from outflow obstruction, such as hesitancy, weak flow, urinary retention and overflow incontinence

**PCPT:** Prostate Cancer Prevention Trial

**PLESS:** Proscar Long-term Efficacy and Safety Study

**PSA:** prostate-specific antigen, a glycoprotein secreted by the prostate that acts as a marker for prostate disease

**PVF:** post-void residual urine

**SMART-1**: Symptom Management After Reducing Therapy study

**Stents:** mesh-like structures inserted into the prostatic urethra to maintain patency

**TRUS:** transrectal ultrasonography

**TUIP:** transurethral incision of the prostate

**TUMT:** transurethral microwave thermotherapy

**TUNA:** transurethral needle ablation

**TURP:** transurethral resection of the prostate

**VLAP:** visual laser ablation of the prostate (also called ELAP)

# Introduction

Benign prostatic hyperplasia (BPH) is one of the most common diseases to affect men beyond middle age. Histological disease (microscopic BPH) is present in more than 60% of men in their sixties, and over 40% of men beyond this age have lower urinary tract symptoms (LUTS) (Figure 1); about half of this group has an impaired quality of life. The prevalence increases with age, and thus the absolute number of patients affected is rising worldwide as a result of aging populations. At current intervention rates, about one-fifth of patients with symptomatic disease who present to a doctor will eventually be treated surgically. The remainder will often be managed initially by active surveillance ('watchful waiting'). However, the majority of these individuals suffer gradual progression of symptoms and the bother associated with them, and increasingly require treatment either with medication or surgery.

Nowadays, BPH is rarely a life-threatening condition. Deterioration of symptoms and urinary flow is usually slow, and serious outcomes, such as renal insufficiency, are uncommon. The risk of acute urinary

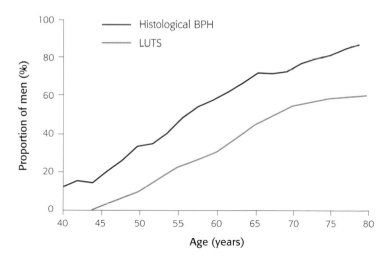

**Figure 1** The incidences of both histological benign prostatic hyperplasia (BPH) and lower urinary tract symptoms (LUTS) increase progressively with age.

retention (AUR), however, increases with prostate size, and requires urgent hospitalization and often surgery. The relatively less serious symptoms of frequency, nocturia and incomplete bladder emptying can nevertheless be very bothersome, and may impact substantially on the patient's quality of life. In addition, men with LUTS due to BPH are also prone to erectile dysfunction (ED) and disorders of ejaculation.

Extensive research into BPH in recent years has resulted not only in a clearer understanding of its pathogenesis, but also in the development of new medical and minimally invasive surgical treatments. At the same time, patients' awareness of prostate disease has grown. Today, therefore, the choice of treatment for BPH requires a balance between several factors:

• clinical need and considerations concerning the prevention of disease progression for the individual
• the preferences of the patient and of his immediate family
• cost–benefit ratio and long-term effectiveness of therapy.

Treatment that carries the proven possibility of safely enhancing the quality of life has to be tailored to the affected individual with these factors in mind.

The fifth edition of *Fast Facts – Benign Prostatic Hyperplasia* provides a concise overview of the pathophysiology, diagnosis and treatment of BPH. The latest data on the safety and efficacy of various treatment strategies are included, as well as new preventive considerations. The emphasis is on providing up-to-date practical information that will enable the patient and the primary care physician – who is becoming increasingly involved in the care of the broad spectrum of prostatic diseases – to decide together the nature of the problem and the most appropriate treatment.

**Key references**

Girman CJ, Jacobsen SJ, Rhodes T et al. Association of health-related quality of life and benign prostatic enlargement. *Eur Urol* 1999;35:277–84.

Kirby RS. The natural history of BPH: What have we learned in the last decade? *Urology* 2000;56:3–6.

The prostate consists of three distinct zones (Figure 1.1):
- a central zone
- a peripheral zone
- a transition zone, adjacent to the urethra.

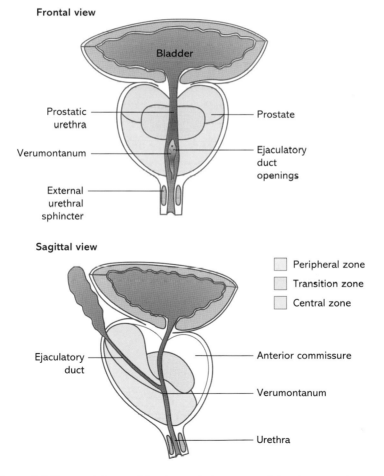

**Frontal view**

Bladder

Prostatic urethra

Prostate

Verumontanum

Ejaculatory duct openings

External urethral sphincter

**Sagittal view**

☐ Peripheral zone
☐ Transition zone
☐ Central zone

Ejaculatory duct

Anterior commissure

Verumontanum

Urethra

**Figure 1.1** The prostate consists of a central zone, a peripheral zone, and a transition zone, the last of which is the usual site of development of BPH.

BPH develops almost exclusively in the transition zone, whereas prostate cancer usually develops in the peripheral zone.

## Pathogenesis of BPH

The growth and development of the prostate is under the influence of the male hormone testosterone and its more active metabolite dihydrotestosterone (DHT). The enzyme $5\alpha$-reductase ($5\alpha$-R) is responsible for the conversion of testosterone to DHT. It has two isoforms: type 2 $5\alpha$-R predominates in the prostate, whereas both type 1 and type 2 $5\alpha$-R are common in extraprostatic tissues. BPH requires DHT stimulation of androgen receptors; this results in the transcription and translation of growth factors, such as epidermal growth factor (EGF). This in turn promotes the stromal and epithelial hyperplasia characteristic of BPH. Other factors underlying the hyperplastic process include a reduction in programmed cell death (apoptosis). Transforming growth factor $\beta$ (TGF$\beta$) is one of the factors involved in this process. Imbalance between molecules stimulating proliferation and those inducing apoptosis results in progressive hyperplastic enlargement of the transition zone of the prostate (Figure 1.2).

Although BPH is often thought to be the result of glandular proliferation, in fact up to 60% of hyperplastic tissue is composed of smooth muscle cells and connective tissue. Contraction of these smooth muscle cells is under the control of the sympathetic nervous system. When noradrenaline is released from dense core vesicles contained within the sympathetic nerve terminal, it diffuses across the synaptic gap to bind to numerous $\alpha_1$-adrenoceptors located on the membrane of prostatic smooth muscle cells. The resultant influx of calcium increases prostatic smooth muscle tone. Several $\alpha_1$-adrenoceptor subtypes are known. The $\alpha_{1A}$-subtype is the predominant receptor in the prostate, while the $\alpha_{1B}$-subtype seems to be mainly involved in peripheral vasoconstriction, and the $\alpha_{1D}$-adrenoceptors appear to exist mainly in the liver, spleen and bladder. As a result of these observations, there has been considerable interest in developing pharmacological agents that are highly $\alpha_{1A}$-selective in their activity, although there is now some doubt about how effective these will be clinically.

## Pathology of BPH

The first histological sign of BPH, which may occur even in men in their forties, is the appearance of stromal nodules in the periurethral area of the transition zone. The nodules vary in size from a few millimeters to a few centimeters. Nodule formation is followed by glandular hyperplasia. Unlike clinical (symptomatic) BPH, the incidence of pathological BPH is very similar in all populations that have been studied.

Rather surprisingly, there is no very close correlation between the overall size of the prostate and the degree of outflow obstruction. There are a number of factors that may account for this:

- the relative proportions of stromal and glandular tissue in the prostate
- variations in sympathetic nervous stimulation of prostatic smooth muscle
- variable enlargement of the middle lobe of the prostate, leading to 'ball-valve' obstruction without overall enlargement of the gland
- variations in the response of the bladder to obstruction and aging.

However, the larger the prostate, the greater is the risk of BPH

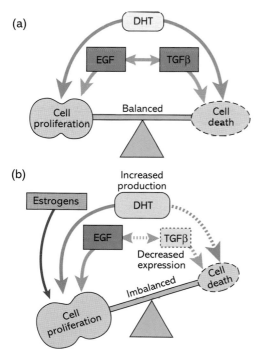

Figure 1.2 (a) In the normal prostate, cell formation is balanced by programmed cell death (apoptosis). (b) BPH develops when growth factors such as epidermal growth factor (EGF) promote excessive cell division or when lack of transforming growth factor β (TGFβ) reduces the rate of cell death. DHT, dihydrotestosterone.

progression and complications such as acute urinary retention and the need for surgery.

## Role of prostate-specific antigen

Prostate-specific antigen (PSA) is a glycoprotein protease secreted by prostatic epithelial cells that liquefies semen after ejaculation. Its secretion is often increased in patients with BPH (Figure 1.3). On average, serum PSA levels have been reported to increase by 0.3 ng/mL per gram of BPH tissue; however, much larger increases are usually seen in patients with clinical prostate cancer. Elevated serum PSA levels (> 4.0 ng/mL) occur in about 25% or more of men with BPH, and in most patients with prostate cancer of significant volume. Therefore, PSA is not a diagnostic test for prostate cancer, but does afford an estimate of the probability of the presence of prostate cancer (this, and the use of free:total PSA ratio, is discussed on pages 26–9). In addition, it provides a useful surrogate estimate for prostate volume, since in

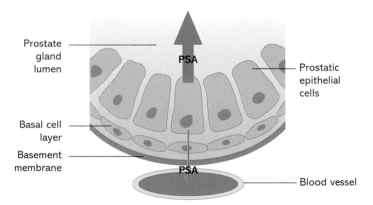

**Figure 1.3** Prostate-specific antigen (PSA) is secreted from epithelial cells of the prostate and constitutes an important component of prostatic secretions. Normally only a small proportion is absorbed into the bloodstream. Conditions that disrupt the basal cell layer, such as prostate cancer, result in increased absorption and elevated serum PSA values. BPH can also cause a moderate elevation of PSA. In the absence of cancer, the serum PSA value can provide a useful surrogate estimate of prostate volume.

BPH the larger the gland, in general, the higher the PSA level (specifically, a higher PSA value predicts a greater number of actively secreting epithelial cells, Figure 1.4). This is of clinical value, since men with larger prostates are at significantly greater risk of disease progression than those with smaller glands.

## Natural history of BPH

BPH is usually a slowly progressive condition; longitudinal population-based studies have shown an average decline in peak urine flow rate of about 0.2 mL/second/year and an average increase in prostate volume of 1–2 cm³/year. Recently it has been reported that there is some variability between individuals in the rate of prostate growth; in general those with larger glands tend to suffer faster prostate growth rates. This is not, however, always accompanied by progressive worsening of symptoms, which may be explained partly by the fact that BPH symptoms sometimes fluctuate considerably. Symptoms may remain stable or even improve with time in some individuals (Figure 1.5), and patients often make lifestyle adjustments for the disorder by, for example, restricting their fluid intake. Nevertheless, BPH negatively affects quality of life and may be associated with sexual dysfunction.

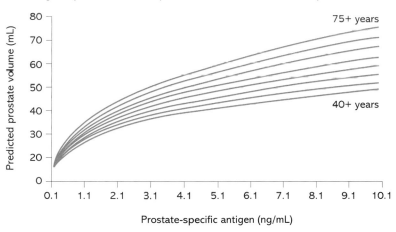

Figure 1.4 Estimated prostate volume as a function of serum PSA value at 5-year intervals, from 40+ years (the lowest curve) to 75+ years (highest). Reproduced from Mochtar et al., copyright © 2003, with permisison from the European Association of Urology.

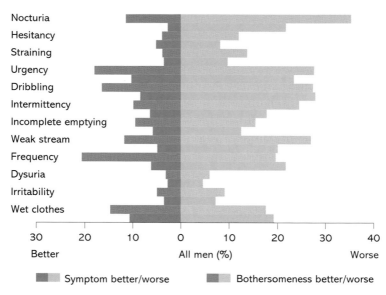

Figure 1.5 The symptoms of BPH may remain unchanged or deteriorate slowly. Reproduced from Lee et al. 1996 with permission from S Karger AG, Basel.

**Early disease.** As BPH progresses, the gland enlarges, and normal prostatic tissue becomes increasingly compressed by hyperplastic tissue. This impinges upon the prostatic urethra (Figure 1.6), which, in turn, becomes less distensible, causing progressive obstruction of urine flow. Patients complain of hesitancy, a reduced stream and incomplete bladder emptying. The detrusor muscle responds to this obstruction by smooth muscle hypertrophy and connective tissue infiltration, resulting in increased voiding pressures, decreased bladder compliance and involuntary bladder contractions (detrusor overactivity) in up to 70%

TABLE 1.1

**Causes of nocturnal polyuria**

- Congestive cardiac failure
- Antidiuretic hormone disturbance
- Sleep disturbance
- Excessive evening fluid intake

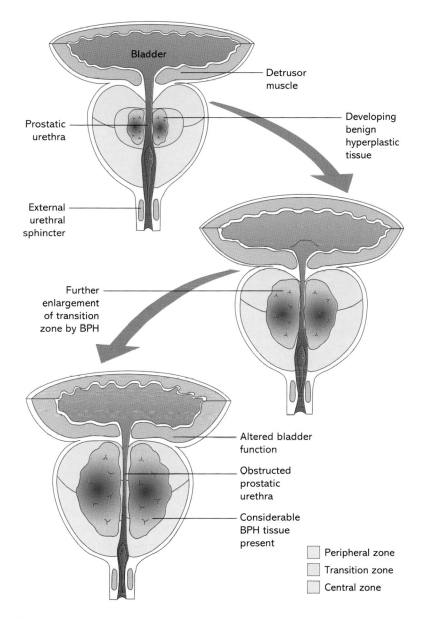

**Figure 1.6** As BPH progresses, hyperplastic tissue progressively encroaches on the prostatic urethra, resulting in gradual obstruction of urinary flow and secondary changes in bladder function caused by smooth muscle hypertrophy, changes in the extracellular matrix and neuronal alterations.

15

of patients. Secondary detrusor overactivity may occur as a result of obstruction-induced changes to the nervous system, and this might explain the irritative LUTS of BPH, such as frequency, urgency and nocturia. However, LUTS may also be a result of unrelated conditions such as nocturnal polyuria (Table 1.1), urinary tract infection, tuberculosis, carcinoma in situ, bladder stones or neurogenic bladder dysfunction. These differential diagnoses need to be borne in mind when treatment is selected.

**Advanced disease.** Progressive impairment of bladder emptying may culminate in acute urinary retention (AUR), a distressing condition requiring urgent catheterization and often hospitalization. If gradual overdistension occurs, painless retention may result in enuresis, in addition to the usual LUTS (see Table 2.2, page 22). In severe cases, the degree of bladder overdistension may preclude full recovery of bladder function. Risk factors for AUR have recently been defined (Table 1.2). Men with enlarged prostates are more likely than those with small prostates to develop acute retention or need prostate surgery.

Although uncommon, prolonged outflow obstruction can also cause:
- bladder stone formation (Figure 1.7)
- formation of bladder diverticula (Figure 1.8)
- recurrent urinary tract infections
- chronic urinary retention
- deterioration of renal function (rare).

TABLE 1.2

**Risk factors for acute urinary retention**

- Age of patient (risk increases with age)
- Large hyperplastic prostate
- High PSA values
- Increased post-void residual urine
- Reduced urinary flow rate ($Q_{max}$ < 10 mL/s)
- Previous history of acute urinary retention
- Severe lower urinary tract symptoms

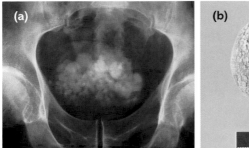
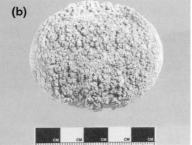

Figure 1.7 (a) A plain abdominal radiograph showing stones in situ.
(b) Outflow obstruction may result in the formation of a bladder stone.

## Factors influencing the development of BPH

The only clearly defined risk factors for BPH are age and the presence
of androgens secreted by functioning testes. Other factors, however,
may influence the prevalence of clinical disease.

Race and environment. Clinical BPH has been reported to be more
common in Western societies. Asian races appear to have a lower
incidence than white races, and there is some evidence that Asians who
migrate to Western countries increase their risk of developing BPH,
suggesting that environmental factors are also involved. As westernized
diets are adopted in countries such as Japan, so the incidence of BPH
appears to be rising.

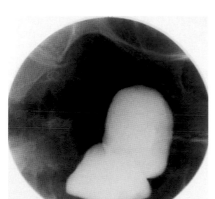

Figure 1.8 A large diverticulum
caused by prolonged bladder outflow
obstruction.

17

**Diet.** BPH has been reported to be less common in men who eat large amounts of vegetables. It has been suggested that certain vegetables protect against BPH because they contain phytoestrogens, such as genistein, which have antiandrogenic effects on the prostate. This may account for reported differences in incidence of BPH between East and West, but hard data supporting this theory have yet to be produced.

**Genetics.** Clinical BPH seems to run in families. If one or more first-degree relatives have been affected, then the individual is at greater risk of being afflicted by the disorder.

## Changing terminology in BPH

It is now appreciated that BPH is in fact a pathological rather than a clinical diagnosis. LUTS may or may not be due to BPH; similarly, bladder outflow obstruction (BOO) may or may not be present. The three interrelated components of the disease are illustrated in Figure 1.9. When all three are present then the patient is at greatest risk of disease progression.

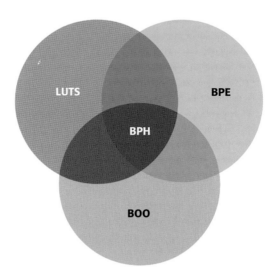

**Figure 1.9** The three components of BPH – benign prostatic enlargement (BPE), lower urinary tract symptoms (LUTS) and bladder outflow obstruction (BOO) – may occur independently or, commonly, together.

## Key points – pathophysiology of BPH

- BPH is a gradually progressive condition.
- Prostate enlargement often results in symptoms and bladder outflow obstruction.
- Men with larger prostates (and higher PSA values) are at greater risk of complications such as AUR and the need for surgery.
- BPH can negatively affect quality of life and may be associated with sexual dysfunction.

### Key references

Arrighi H, Guess H, Metter E, Fozard J. Symptoms and signs of prostatism as risk factors for prostatectomy. *Prostate* 1990;16:253–61.

Ball AJ, Feneley RCL, Abrams PH. The natural history of untreated 'prostatism'. *Br J Urol* 1981;533: 613–16.

Berry SJ, Coffey DS, Walsh PC, Ewing LL. The development of human benign prostatic hyperplasia with age. *J Urol* 1984;132:474–9.

Ekman P. BPH epidemiology and risk factors. *Prostate* 1989;2(suppl):23–31.

Garraway WM, Kirby RS. Benign prostatic hyperplasia: effects on quality of life and impact on treatment decisions. *Urology* 1994;44:629–36.

Garraway WM, McKelvie GB, Russell EBAW et al. Impact of previously unrecognised benign prostatic hyperplasia on the daily activities of middle-aged and elderly men. *Br J Gen Pract* 1993;43:318–21.

Girman CJ, Epstein RS, Jacobsen SJ et al. Natural history of prostatism: impact of urinary symptoms on quality of life in 2115 randomly selected community men. *Urology* 1994;44:825–31.

Glynn RJ, Campion EW, Bouchard GR, Silbert JE. The development of benign prostatic hyperplasia among volunteers in the normative aging study. *Am J Epidemiol* 1985;121:78–90.

Isaacs JT, Coffey DS. Etiology and disease process of benign prostatic hyperplasia. *Prostate* 1989;2(suppl):33–50.

Lee AJ, Russell EB, Garraway WM, Prescott RJ. Three-year follow-up of a community-based cohort of men with untreated benign prostatic hyperplasia. *Eur Urol* 1996;30: 11–17.

Lukacs B, Comet D, Doublet D et al. Two-year assessment of long-term Health-Related Quality of Life (HRQL) of 4591 patients suffering from benign prostatic hypertrophy (BPH) treated with a uro-selective alpha-1 blocker, alfuzosin. *J Urol* 1996;155:574A.

Mochtar CA, Kiemeney LALM, van Riemsdijk MM et al. Prostate-specific antigen as an estimator of prostate volume in the management of patients with symptomatic benign prostatic hyperplasia. *Eur Urol* 2003;44:695–700.

Roehrborn CG, Schwinn DA. Alpha1-adrenergic receptors and their inhibitors in lower urinary tract symptoms and benign prostatic hyperplasia. *J Urol* 2004;171: 1029–35.

BPH is the most prevalent condition affecting the prostate, accounting for over 80% of clinical presentations for prostate disease. Patients in whom BPH is suspected, or who simply require reassurance that they do not have a prostate disorder, should undergo a basic evaluation (Table 2.1).

## History and symptom assessment

BPH is characterized by a spectrum of obstructive and irritative symptoms, known collectively as LUTS (Table 2.2). It should be remembered, however, that these symptoms are not specific to BPH and may also occur in patients with prostate cancer, prostatitis or other disorders. Poor urinary flow and the sensation of incomplete bladder emptying are the two symptoms that correlate most closely with the eventual need for prostate surgery. Dribbling after micturition is usually due to pooling of urine in the bulbar urethra rather than obstruction. The history should focus on the urinary tract and general health issues, as well as fitness for surgery. Conditions such as Parkinson's disease or stroke, polyuria from diabetes or congestive heart failure, history of urethral strictures, or treatment with, for example, anticholinergic or antidepressant drugs should be excluded as causes of similar urinary symptoms (Table 2.3). LUTS have been shown to constitute an

TABLE 2.1

**Basic evaluation of BPH**

- Detailed history and symptom assessment
- Physical examination, including digital rectal examination
- Urinalysis
- Measurement of serum prostate-specific antigen (optional, but should be considered in men with at least a 10-year life expectancy and for whom management would be changed by a diagnosis of prostate cancer)

TABLE 2.2

**Lower urinary tract symptoms associated with BPH\***

**Obstructive (storage) symptoms**

- Hesitancy
- Weak stream
- Straining to pass urine
- Prolonged micturition
- Feeling of incomplete bladder emptying
- Acute urinary retention
- Nocturnal enuresis due to chronic retention

**Irritative (voiding) symptoms**

- Frequency
- Urgency
- Nocturia
- Urge incontinence

\*The value of categorizing symptoms into obstructive and irritative is questioned by some experts.

TABLE 2.3

**Differential diagnosis of lower urinary tract symptoms**

**Neurological conditions**

- Parkinson's disease
- Cerebrovascular accident
- Multiple system atrophy (Shy–Drager syndrome)
- Cerebral atrophy
- Multiple sclerosis
- Sleep apnea

**Inflammatory disorders**

- Urinary tract infection/ bladder stone
- Interstitial cystitis
- Tuberculous cystitis

**Neoplastic disorders**

- Prostate cancer
- Carcinoma in situ of the bladder

**Causes of polyuria**

- Diabetes
- Congestive heart failure
- Excessive fluid intake

**Other causes of obstruction**

- Bladder neck dyssynergia
- External sphincter dyssynergia
- Urethral stricture
- Severe phimosis

independent risk factor for sexual dysfunction in older men. Since sexual dysfunction is associated with impaired quality of life and is readily treatable, men presenting with BPH should be specifically asked about the presence or absence of this problem.

The frequency of symptoms can be assessed quantitatively by means of the International Prostate Symptom Score (IPSS) or American

| | Not at all | Less than 1 time in 5 | Less than half the time | About half the time | More than half the time | Almost always |
|---|---|---|---|---|---|---|
| | | | | **Patient score** | | |
| **● Incomplete emptying**<br>Over the past month, how often have you had a sensation of not emptying your bladder completely after you finished urinating? | 0 | 1 | 2 | 3 | 4 | 5 |
| **● Frequency**<br>Over the past month, how often have you had to urinate again less than 2 hours after you finished urinating? | 0 | 1 | 2 | 3 | 4 | 5 |
| **● Intermittency**<br>Over the past month, how often have you found you stopped and started again several times when you urinated? | 0 | 1 | 2 | 3 | 4 | 5 |
| **● Urgency**<br>Over the past month, how often have you found it difficult to postpone urination? | 0 | 1 | 2 | 3 | 4 | 5 |
| **● Weak stream**<br>Over the past month, how often have you had a weak urinary stream? | 0 | 1 | 2 | 3 | 4 | 5 |
| **● Straining**<br>Over the past month, how often have you had to push or strain to begin urination? | 0 | 1 | 2 | 3 | 4 | 5 |
| | | | | **Number of times** | | |
| **● Nocturia**<br>Over the past month, how many times did you most typically get up to urinate from the time you went to bed at night until the time you got up in the morning? | 0 | 1 | 2 | 3 | 4 | 5+ |
| **Total IPSS** | | | | | | |

**Figure 2.1** The International Prostate Symptom Score (IPSS) is an important aspect of the initial evaluation in patients with suspected BPH.

Urological Association (AUA) Symptom Score Index (Figure 2.1). These symptom scores are identical and consist of seven questions relating to the severity of symptoms. The maximum possible score is 35; scores of 0–8 are generally regarded as mild, 9–19 as moderate, and 20 or above as severe. A further four questions evaluate the 'bothersomeness' of the symptoms. This is known as the BPH Impact Index (BII) (Figure 2.2) and carries a maximum score of 13. The IPSS and AUA scores are used to measure symptom severity only, and are not diagnostic tests to determine whether symptoms are due to BPH.

## The physical examination

A digital rectal examination (DRE) should form the cornerstone of the physical examination of patients with BPH. DRE provides useful information about the size, consistency and anatomical limits of the

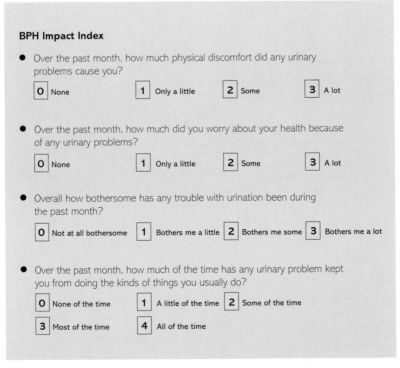

**BPH Impact Index**

- Over the past month, how much physical discomfort did any urinary problems cause you?

  | **0** None | **1** Only a little | **2** Some | **3** A lot |

- Over the past month, how much did you worry about your health because of any urinary problems?

  | **0** None | **1** Only a little | **2** Some | **3** A lot |

- Overall how bothersome has any trouble with urination been during the past month?

  | **0** Not at all bothersome | **1** Bothers me a little | **2** Bothers me some | **3** Bothers me a lot |

- Over the past month, how much of the time has any urinary problem kept you from doing the kinds of things you usually do?

  | **0** None of the time | **1** A little of the time | **2** Some of the time |

  | **3** Most of the time | **4** All of the time |

**Figure 2.2** The BPH Impact Index (BII) quantifies how much the symptoms of BPH bother a patient.

prostate (Table 2.4) and can be performed with the patient in the left lateral (Figure 2.3) or knee–elbow position. Studies suggest that DRE provides a reasonably accurate estimation of volume in prostates of 50 cm³ or less. However, the volume of larger glands tends to be underestimated by this technique.

In addition to DRE, the abdomen should be examined to detect a palpable bladder due to chronic urinary retention. The physical examination should also include a focused neurological examination, together with some specific enquiries, to exclude disorders of the nervous system, such as a cauda equina lesion or Parkinson's disease, as the underlying cause of the patient's symptoms.

## Urinalysis

Ideally, urinalysis – either by dipstick or by microscopic examination of sediment – should be performed in all men presenting with LUTS. Such investigations help to distinguish BPH from urinary tract infection or bladder cancer, which may produce symptoms similar to those of BPH. If the dipstick result is positive, urine microscopy and culture should be performed and further imaging and evaluation of the renal tract considered. Urine cytology should be requested in those with severely irritative symptoms to exclude a diagnosis of carcinoma in situ of the

TABLE 2.4

**DRE provides useful clinical information for the diagnosis of BPH**

| | |
|---|---|
| Size | The normal prostate is slightly smaller than a golf ball (20 cm³). In patients with BPH, it may exceed the size of a tennis ball (> 50 cm³). |
| Consistency | The benign gland feels smooth, symmetrical and elastic; a palpable nodule or a diffusely hardened and asymmetric gland may indicate cancer. |
| Anatomical limits | The lateral and cranial borders and the median sulcus of the prostate should be identifiable. The seminal vesicles should be impalpable; hardening suggests invasion by prostate cancer. |

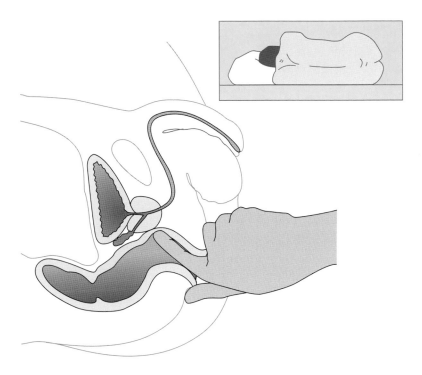

**Figure 2.3** Digital rectal examination of the prostate should be performed carefully and the results recorded for all patients with lower urinary tract symptoms.

bladder. If urine cytology is positive an intravenous urogram (IVU) and lower tract endoscopy and biopsy are mandatory.

## Prostate-specific antigen

Although PSA determination is an optional test, it should be seriously considered for all men with a life expectancy of 10 years or more, for whom identification of prostate cancer would influence treatment decisions (Tables 2.5 and 2.6). Measurement of PSA increases the likelihood of detecting prostate cancer over and above DRE alone and is most relevant, therefore, in such men, who are most likely to benefit. Overall, if PSA levels are above the upper limit of normal (i.e. 4.0 ng/mL), the likelihood of prostate cancer is about 20–25%. If PSA is considerably elevated (> 10 ng/mL), the likelihood of cancer rises

TABLE 2.5

Interpretation of prostate-specific antigen (PSA) levels alone

| PSA level (mg/mL) | Interpretation |
| --- | --- |
| < 4 | Normal, unless rising by > 25%/year |
| 4–10 | 20–25% chance of cancer – consider biopsy |
| > 10 | > 50% chance of cancer – biopsy usually indicated |
| Rise of > 0.75 ng/mL/year | Refer urgently for evaluation |

TABLE 2.6

Percentage risk of prostate cancer using a combination of prostate-specific antigen (PSA) level and digital rectal examination (DRE) results

| | PSA (ng/mL) | | |
| --- | --- | --- | --- |
| | < 4 | 4–10 | > 10 |
| Negative DRE | 9% | 20% | 31% |
| Positive DRE | 17% | 45% | 77% |

to over 50%. In general, the higher the PSA, the greater the chance of malignancy. It is often not possible, however, to distinguish men with localized prostate cancer from those with BPH on the basis of a single PSA measurement without recourse to a transrectal ultrasound-guided prostatic biopsy, and patients should be informed of this.

It has also become apparent that in the absence of prostate cancer, measurement of serum PSA values can provide a useful indication of overall prostate volume. This, in turn, can predict those patients most likely to suffer BPH progression and in turn facilitate the selection of agents for medical therapy of BPH. Not surprisingly, men with enlarged prostates and high PSA values (arbitrarily set as volume > 30 cm$^3$ and PSA value > 1.4 ng/mL) appear to benefit most from 5α-reductase inhibitors, which act primarily by reducing the prostate volume.

Recently, it has been discovered that PSA in the circulation exists in two forms: a 'bound' form, which is complexed to one of two proteins – either antichymotrypsin or $\alpha_2$-macroglobulin – and a 'free' or uncomplexed form (Figure 2.4). For reasons that are not fully understood, the ratio of free:total PSA declines in patients harboring prostate malignancy. Moreover, the more biologically aggressive the tumor appears to be, the greater the reduction in the free:total PSA ratio. Although there is still debate concerning the cut-off point for the free:total PSA ratio, patients with a total PSA level above 4.0 ng/mL and a free:total PSA ratio below 0.18 should usually be referred and considered for prostatic biopsy.

**The screening debate.** One of the most hotly contested issues in medicine at present is screening for prostate cancer. Those advocating population screening point out that early detection by PSA testing, in

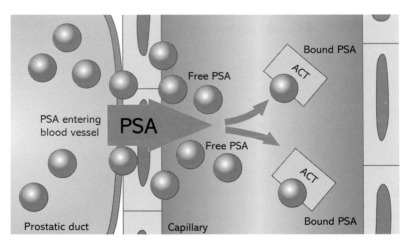

**Figure 2.4** Prostate-specific antigen (PSA) is a glycoprotein released from the epithelial cells of the prostate. In normal men, only small amounts (< 4.0 ng/mL) enter the circulation, where around one-fifth or less is bound to proteins such as antichymotrypsin (ACT). In prostate cancer, large amounts (> 4.0 ng/mL) enter the circulation and a greater proportion is bound to ACT, resulting in a reduced free:total PSA ratio. Patients with BPH usually have only minor elevations of serum PSA values (moderate amounts of PSA enter the circulation, and a small proportion is bound to ACT).

combination with DRE, identifies cancers that are confined to the gland and therefore potentially curable in 70–80% of cases. Critics, however, maintain that many of the cancers diagnosed would never have become clinically manifest within the patient's natural lifespan. As yet no screening-related reduction in prostate-cancer-specific mortality has been definitively demonstrated, and the debate is likely to continue until the results of ongoing randomized studies of screening in Europe and the USA are available. Nonetheless, in the USA, where more than 50% of men routinely have PSA tests, a reduction in mortality from prostate cancer is now being reported.

## Uroflowmetry

Electronic measurement of urine flow rates is an extremely useful non-invasive test in most patients with BPH (Figure 2.5). It is helpful in identifying patients whose peak flow rate is not diminished, and thus are very unlikely to benefit from surgery. Such patients are more likely to be suffering from an overactive bladder than BPH.

Uroflowmetry measures a number of parameters of obstruction, of which the most important is the peak flow rate. A peak flow rate below 15 mL/second (with a voided volume of at least 150 mL) suggests obstruction (Table 2.7), although in older men (70–80 years of age), values of 10–15 mL/second may be normal. The presence of a markedly reduced peak flow rate (< 10 mL/second) usually indicates some degree of obstruction, which is most often caused by BPH; uroflowmetry cannot, of course, distinguish between obstruction and impaired detrusor function as the cause of a low flow rate. In general, those men with severe impairment of urine flow (< 10 mL/second) more often suffer disease progression and eventually require medical or surgical intervention.

## Measurement of residual urine

Measurement of post-void residual (PVR) urine is also a useful optional test in the evaluation of BPH, as it can identify patients who are likely to respond less well to active surveillance (watchful waiting) or medical therapy. In general, PVR values above 200–300 mL usually indicate a higher likelihood of the need for invasive therapy and also a higher risk

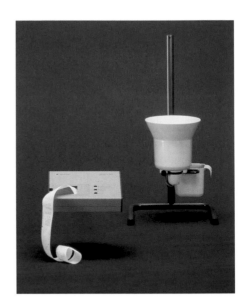

**Figure 2.5** Uroflowmetry using a flowmeter (right) measures a number of parameters of obstruction (below) that are usually altered in patients with BPH.

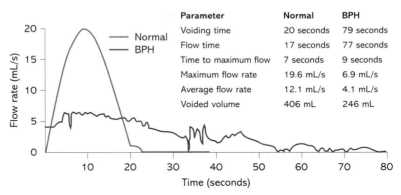

| Parameter | Normal | BPH |
|---|---|---|
| Voiding time | 20 seconds | 79 seconds |
| Flow time | 17 seconds | 77 seconds |
| Time to maximum flow | 7 seconds | 9 seconds |
| Maximum flow rate | 19.6 mL/s | 6.9 mL/s |
| Average flow rate | 12.1 mL/s | 4.1 mL/s |
| Voided volume | 406 mL | 246 mL |

TABLE 2.7

**Interpretation of peak urine flow rates**

| Flow rate (mL/s) | Interpretation |
|---|---|
| > 15 | Unlikely to be obstructed |
| 10–15 | Equivocal |
| < 10 | Either obstructed or weak bladder contractility |

of AUR. The test cannot, however, be used to confirm or exclude BPH. It may be useful as a safety measure in monitoring the progress of patients who opt for active surveillance.

It is best to measure PVR non-invasively by transabdominal ultrasound (Figure 2.6); less commonly, catheterization is used. However, there is considerable void-to-void variation, and thus treatment decisions should not be based on a single measurement alone. Those patients with a consistently high PVR (> 300 mL) should usually be referred for further evaluation and consideration for eventual transurethral surgery.

## Pressure/flow measurements

Pressure/flow measurements (or urodynamics), which involve introducing a small catheter – either urethrally or suprapubically – to measure pressure within the bladder, can be used to distinguish outflow obstruction from impaired detrusor contractility. The routine use of this test in BPH is, however, not indicated. The method is invasive, and inevitably causes some degree of discomfort to the

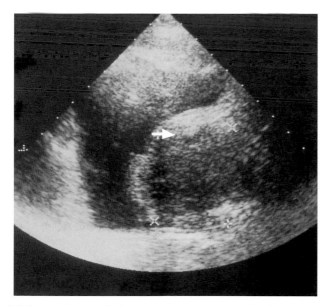

**Figure 2.6** A transabdominal ultrasound scan showing post-void residual urine and a benignly enlarged prostate bulging into the bladder (arrowed).

patient. The current consensus is that this investigation should be confined primarily to those patients with equivocal findings in whom invasive therapy is being considered, as, in the absence of demonstrable obstruction, surgery is not usually appropriate. If urodynamic assessment is recommended, patients should be informed of the pros and cons of the investigation.

## Transrectal ultrasonography

Transrectal ultrasonography (TRUS) is indicated when DRE findings and/or PSA values suggest the possibility of prostate cancer; it also serves to guide the automatic prostate biopsy needle (Figure 2.7). In addition, it can be used to determine prostate volume, which, as already noted, may provide prognostic information and facilitate treatment

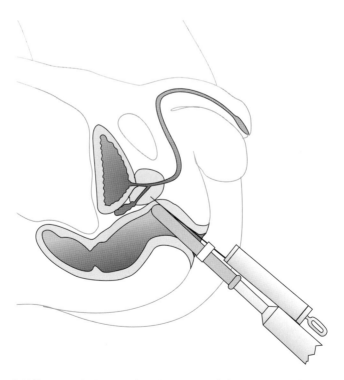

**Figure 2.7** Transrectal ultrasound-guided biopsy of the prostate with an automated biopsy device.

decisions. TRUS should not, however, be regarded as a standard investigation for all patients with bladder outflow obstruction due to BPH.

## Summary of guidelines for diagnosis and management of BPH

A flow chart for the diagnosis and management of BPH is shown in Figure 2.8. Patients presenting with LUTS, or who are identified by asking relevant questions from the IPSS, or who are simply seeking reassurance, should be evaluated using the following criteria:
• a detailed history and assessment of symptoms
• a physical examination, including a DRE
• dipstick urinalysis (and urine microscopy/culture if positive).

In addition, PSA determination should be considered in men with a life expectancy of at least 10 years.

Referral to a urologist is appropriate if the patient has:
• a markedly elevated symptom score, a high BII or very reduced flow rate
• a history of hematuria, urinary retention or recurrent urinary tract infections
• abnormalities detected by DRE, or a palpable bladder
• PSA above 4.0 ng/mL
• free:total PSA ratio below 0.19 (if PSA is in the range of 4–20 ng/mL).

---

**Key points – diagnosis of BPH**

• BPH symptoms can be quantified with the IPSS.
• Physical examination should involve a DRE.
• PSA measurement helps to estimate the risk of prostate cancer and provides a surrogate indication of prostate volume.
• Uroflowmetry helps estimate the severity of obstruction.
• PVR volume (with some variability) reveals voiding efficiency.
• Urodynamics may be helpful in selected cases.

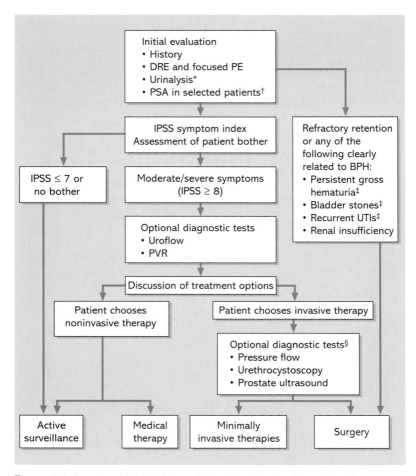

**Figure 2.8** American Urological Association algorithm for diagnosis and management of BPH. *In patients with clinically significant prostatic bleeding, a course of a 5α-reductase inhibitor may be used. If bleeding persists, tissue ablative surgery is indicated. †Patients with at least a 10-year life expectancy for whom knowledge of the presence of prostate cancer would change management of voiding symptoms. ‡After exhausting other therapeutic options. §Some diagnostic tests are used in predicting response to therapy. Pressure–flow studies are most useful in men prior to surgery. DRE, digital rectal examination; IPSS, International Prostate Symptoms Score; PE, physical examination; PSA, prostate-specific antigen; PVR, post-void residual urine; UTI, urinary tract infection. Adapted with permission from the American Urological Association. AUA guideline on management of benign prostatic hyperplasia (2003). *J Urol* 2003;170:530–47.

## Key references

Abrams PH, Griffiths DJ. The assessment of prostatic obstruction from urodynamic measurements and from residual urine. *Br J Urol* 1979;51:129–34.

Abrams PH. Prostatism and prostatectomy: the value of urine flow rate measurement in the preoperative assessment for operation. *J Urol* 1977;117:70–1.

Barry MJ, Fowler FJ, O'Leary MP et al. Correlation of the American Urological Association symptom index with self administered versions of the Madsen–Iversen, Boyarsky, and Maine Medical Assessment Program symptom indexes. *J Urol* 1992;148: 1558–63.

Barry MJ, Fowler FJ, O'Leary MP et al. The American Urological Association symptom index for benign prostatic hyperplasia. *J Urol* 1992;148:1549–57.

Benson MC, Whang IS, Panteuck A et al. Prostate specific antigen density: a means of distinguishing between benign prostatic hypertrophy and prostate cancer. *J Urol* 1992;147: 815–16.

Birch NC, Hurst G, Doyle PT. Serial residual volumes in men with prostatic hypertrophy. *Br J Urol* 1988;62:571–5.

Brawer MK, Chetner MP, Beattie J et al. Screening for prostate cancer with prostate specific antigen. *J Urol* 1992;147:841–5.

Bruskewitz RC, Iversen P, Madsen PO. Value of postvoid residual urine determination in evaluation of prostatism. *Urology* 1982;20:602–4.

Carter BH, Pearson JD, Metter J et al. Longitudinal evaluation of prostate specific antigen levels in men with and without prostate cancer. *JAMA* 1993;267:2215–20.

Catalona WJ, Smith DS, Ratliff TL et al. Measurement of prostate specific antigen in serum as a screening test for prostate cancer. *N Engl J Med* 1991;324: 1156–61.

Chancellor MB, Blaivas JG, Kaplan SA, Axelrod S. Bladder outlet obstruction versus impaired detrusor contractility: the role of uroflow. *J Urol* 1991;145:810–12.

Chisholm GD, Carne SJ, Fitzpatrick JM et al. Prostate disease: management options for the primary health team. *Postgrad Med J* 1995; 71:136–42.

Crawford ED, Schutz MJ, Clejan S et al. The effect of digital rectal examination on prostate specific antigen levels. *JAMA* 1992;267: 2227–8.

Drach GW, Layton TN, Binard WJ. Male peak urinary flow rate: relationship of volume voided and age. *J Urol* 1979;122:210–14.

Gleason DM, Bottaccini MR, Drach GW, Layton TN. Urinary flow velocity as an index of male voiding function. *J Urol* 1982;128:1363–7.

Grino PB, Bruskewitz R, Blaivas JG et al. Maximum urinary flow rate by uroflowmetry: automatic or visual interpretation. *J Urol* 1993;149: 339–41.

Hald T. Urodynamics in benign prostatic hyperplasia: a survey. *Prostate* 1989;2(suppl):69–77.

Jensen KME, Jorgensen JB, Mogensen P. Urodynamics in prostatism I. Prognostic value of uroflowmetry. *Scand J Urol Nephrol* 1988;22:109–17.

Jensen KME, Jorgensen JB, Mogensen P. Urodynamics in prostatism II. Prognostic value of pressure-flow study combined with stop-flow test. *Scand J Urol Nephrol* 1988;114(suppl):72–7.

Kirby RS, Chisholm G, Chapple CR et al. Shared care between general practitioners and urologists in the management of BPH: a survey of attitudes among clinicians. *J R Soc Med* 1995;88:284–8.

Kirby RS, Christmas T. *Benign Prostatic Hyperplasia*. 2nd edn. London: Mosby, 1997.

Kirby RS, Fitzpatrick J, Kirby M, Fitzpatrick A. *Shared Care for Prostatic Diseases*. Oxford: Isis Medical Media, 1994.

Kirby RS, McConnell J, Fitzpatrick J et al. *Textbook of BPH*. Oxford: Isis Medical Media, 1996.

McConnell JD, Barry MJ, Bruskewitz RC et al. *Benign Prostatic Hyperplasia Diagnosis and Treatment. Clinical Practice Guideline No. 8*. AHCPR Publication No. 940582. Rockville, MD: Agency for Health Care Policy and Research, Public Health Service, US Department of Health and Human Sciences, 1994.

Roehrborn CG, Boyle P, Gould L, Waldstreicher J. Serum prostate-specific antigen as a predictor of prostate volume in men with benign prostatic hyperplasia. *Urology* 1999;53:581–9.

Roehrborn CG, Malice M, Cook TJ, Girman CJ. Clinical predictors of spontaneous acute urinary retention in men with LUTS and clinical BPH: a comprehensive analysis of the pooled placebo groups of several large clinical trials. *Urology* 2001:58;210–16.

Roehrborn CG, McConnell JD, Lieber M et al. Serum prostate-specific antigen concentration is a powerful predictor of acute urinary retention and need for surgery in men with clinical benign prostatic hyperplasia. PLESS study group. *Urology* 1999;53:473–80.

Rosen R, Altwein J, Boyle P et al. Lower urinary tract symptoms and male sexual dysfunction: the multinational survey of the ageing male (MSAM-7). *Eur Urol* 2003;44: 637–49.

Schäfer W, Rübben H, Noppeney R, Deutz FJ. Obstructed and unobstructed prostatic obstruction. A plea for urodynamic objectivation of bladder outflow obstruction in benign prostatic hyperplasia. *World J Urol* 1989;6:198–203.

Shoukry I, Susset JG, Elhilali MM, Dutatre D. Role of uroflowmetry in the assessment of lower urinary tract obstruction in adult males. *Br J Urol* 1975;47(Pt 2):559–66.

## 3   Medical management of BPH

Although transurethral resection of the prostate (TURP) is still the benchmark treatment for severely symptomatic and obstructive BPH, a number of alternative therapies have recently been established. The choice of medical or surgical treatment or active surveillance (watchful waiting) should take into account:

- the nature and severity of symptoms
- the extent to which symptoms cause bother and affect the patient's quality of life
- whether urine flow is significantly reduced and associated with an appreciable volume of PVR urine

TABLE 3.1

**Medical treatments for BPH evaluated in placebo-controlled trials**

|  | Agent | Regimen | Time to onset of action |
|---|---|---|---|
| 5$\alpha$-reductase inhibitors | Dutasteride | 0.5 mg once daily | 3–6 months |
|  | Finasteride | 5 mg once daily | 3–6 months |
| $\alpha_1$-blockers | Alfuzosin SR* | 10 mg once daily[†] | 2–4 weeks |
|  | Doxazosin GITS* | 4–8 mg once daily[‡] |  |
|  | Indoramin** | 20 mg twice daily[‡] |  |
|  | Prazosin** | 2 mg twice daily[‡] |  |
|  | Tamsulosin*§ | 0.4 mg once daily[†] |  |
|  | Terazosin* | 5–10 mg once daily[‡] |  |

*Longer-acting.
**Short-acting.
[†]Does not require dose titration.
[‡]Requires dose titration.
§$\alpha_{1A}$-selective.

38

- the volume of the prostate and the PSA value, which help to predict the risk of acute urinary retention and the need for eventual surgery. The two principal evidence-based approaches to the medical management of BPH are treatment with $\alpha_1$-blockers and 5$\alpha$-reductase inhibitors (Table 3.1).

## Selection of patients

Medical management of BPH should be regarded as an option in its own right, rather than merely an interim measure in patients waiting for surgery. It is suitable for most patients with moderate symptoms; several studies have confirmed that severely symptomatic patients (IPSS > 20) may also respond to these drugs. Patients with mild symptoms (IPSS ≤ 8) and little associated bother should usually be managed by active surveillance. Contraindications to medical

| Mechanism of action/benefits | Adverse effects |
| --- | --- |
| • Reduction of prostatic volume<br>• Reversal of BPH process<br>• Reduction of risks of surgical intervention and acute retention in men with enlarged prostate<br>• Reduction of male-pattern balding | • Erectile dysfunction<br>• Decreased libido<br>• Reduced ejaculate volume<br>• Gynecomastia (rare) |
| • Relaxation of prostatic smooth muscle<br>• Relief of obstruction<br>• Reduction of blood pressure in hypertensive patients | • Tiredness or asthenia<br>• Headache<br>• Dizziness, postural hypotension<br>• Occasionally, retrograde or delayed ejaculation; nasal congestion; reflex tachycardia |

Always refer to the manufacturer's prescribing information.

management include recurrent urinary retention and complications of BPH, such as renal insufficiency, bladder stones or recurrent hematuria (Table 3.2).

Before starting medical treatment, patients should undergo basic evaluation (see Table 2.2, page 22). Symptoms should be assessed every 3–6 months during treatment to monitor the patient's response and ensure that no other intervention is required. DRE and serum PSA measurement should ideally be performed every 6–12 months.

## $\alpha_1$-blockers

Selective $\alpha_1$-blockers, such as prazosin, indoramin, alfuzosin, and – more recently – the longer-acting agents terazosin, doxazosin, slow-release alfuzosin (alfuzosin SR) and the $\alpha_{1A}$-selective compound tamsulosin, have all been shown to increase peak urine flow rate and improve symptoms in about 60% of patients with symptomatic BPH. They are of limited value in patients with complete inability to urinate, although a recent study suggests that $\alpha$-blockers may increase the chances of a successful trial without catheter after an episode of acute retention. $\alpha_1$-blockers act by blocking $\alpha_1$-adrenoceptors in prostatic smooth muscle and in the bladder neck (Figure 3.1), thus reducing outflow obstruction without adversely affecting detrusor contractility. With the exception of prazosin and indoramin, they are given once

TABLE 3.2

**Contraindications to medical treatment of BPH**

- Recurrent acute urinary retention (after failed trial of catheter preceded by $\alpha$-blocker therapy)
- Palpable bladder, large volume of post-void residual urine (> 300 mL)
- Renal insufficiency due to BPH
- Recurrent hematuria due to prostatic bleeding
- Recurrent urinary tract infections secondary to BPH
- Bladder stones or diverticula
- Evidence of prostate cancer (although $\alpha$-blockers may still be used as symptomatic therapy)

daily. With modern formulations dose titration is no longer necessary when starting treatment.

**Efficacy.** Controlled trials with $\alpha_1$-blockers have shown mean improvement in symptom scores of about 30–40%. Overall, the probability that an individual will experience significant symptom improvement with $\alpha_1$-blocker treatment is more than 50%. Both obstructive and irritative symptoms improve rapidly during treatment, usually within the first 2–3 weeks; alternative treatment should be considered if no clinical improvement is seen after 3–4 months.

Treatment with $\alpha_1$-blockers also produces a rapid and significant increase in peak urine flow rate on the order of 1.5–3.5 mL/second. Several studies have also reported a small decrease in detrusor pressure during voiding as a result of treatment, indicating a reduction in the

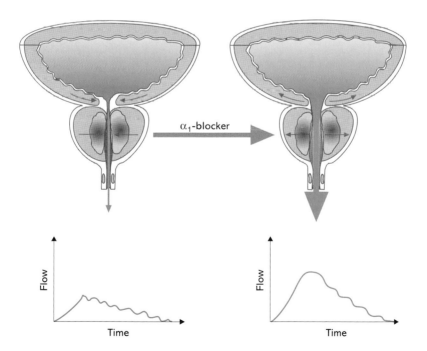

**Figure 3.1** $\alpha_1$-blockers, such as alfuzosin SR, doxazosin and tamsulosin, relax bladder-neck and prostate smooth muscle when used in the treatment of BPH, thereby increasing urinary flow and improving symptoms.

degree of obstruction. Overall, 70–75% of patients continue with $\alpha_1$-blocker therapy.

As yet, relatively few randomized placebo-controlled studies have examined the long-term (> 6 months) use of $\alpha_1$-blockers in patients with BPH. In open-label studies with terazosin, alfuzosin, tamsulosin and doxazosin, lasting up to 4 years, improvements in symptom scores and flow rates seen during the initial treatment period have been maintained during long-term treatment. However, the Medical Treatment of Prostatic Symptoms (MTOPS) study has shown that the $\alpha_1$-blocker doxazosin improves symptoms and delays BPH progression, but does not reduce the risk of AUR or the need for invasive therapy (see Combination therapy, page 49). Certain $\alpha_1$-blockers, such as doxazosin and terazosin, are also recognized as an effective treatment option for hypertension and so may be of particular value in the estimated 25–40% of patients with concomitant obstructive BPH and essential hypertension.

In normotensive patients, doxazosin and terazosin produce only minimal, clinically insignificant blood pressure changes. Doxazosin also appears to affect the lipid profile beneficially by reducing low-density lipoprotein (LDL) cholesterol and triglycerides, and increasing high-density lipoprotein (HDL) cholesterol. These changes could potentially translate into a reduction of risk for cardiovascular disease, such as stroke or myocardial infarction. However, data from the Antihypertensive and Lipid-Lowering treatment to prevent Heart Attack Trial (ALLHAT) suggest that $\alpha_1$-blockers may increase the risk of heart failure, so they should be avoided in hypertensive patients who are at risk of congestive cardiac failure.

Recent data indicate that $\alpha_1$-blockers, particularly alfuzosin and tamsulosin, may reduce the incidence of recurrent AUR after trial without catheter following the inital episode.

**Adverse effects.** The main side effects of $\alpha_1$-blockers result from the cardiovascular and cerebral effects of $\alpha_1$-receptor blockade (Table 3.1). The most common side effects are tiredness, dizziness and headache, occurring in up to 15% of patients. Postural hypotension occurs in only 2–6% of patients, and this may be minimized by using new slow-release formulations and more uroselective agents, persisting with therapy and perhaps taking the medication at night. The incidence of all side effects is lower with the newer, longer-acting agents, and most adverse events tend to diminish with time if the patient is encouraged to continue with medication.

**Uroselectivity.** An area of heated debate is the extent to which side effects can be minimized by the so-called 'uroselectivity' of certain $\alpha_1$-blocking agents. On the basis of clinical and experimental studies, it has been suggested that alfuzosin is more active in the relaxation of prostate-associated, as opposed to cardiovascular-associated, smooth muscle; however, the mechanism is unclear. It has been proposed that tamsulosin exhibits some selectivity for the $\alpha_{1A}$-adrenoceptor subtype (the subtype mainly responsible for prostatic smooth muscle tone), accounting for its minimal effect on blood pressure in either hypertensive or normotensive patients. In one recent study, tamsulosin was better tolerated than terazosin. This has stimulated the quest for even more $\alpha_{1A}$-selective blockers, but none has been approved by the regulatory authorities to date.

**Outcomes.** Although doxazosin has been shown to cause apoptosis in the prostate, there is no evidence currently that $\alpha_1$-blockers prevent the pathological progression of BPH. It has been estimated that treatment will fail within 5 years in 13–39% of patients treated with $\alpha_1$-blockers; this may be comparable to the projected failure rate of active surveillance. In general, further alternative treatments are more likely to be required following medical therapy than after surgical procedures.

## 5α-reductase inhibitors

5α-reductase inhibitors act by inhibiting the enzyme 5α-reductase, which occurs in two forms, 5α-reductase types 1 and 2, and converts testosterone to DHT. As DHT plays a key role in controlling prostate growth, inhibition of these enzymes causes the hyperplasia to regress. Thus, unlike $\alpha_1$-blockers, 5α-reductase inhibitors can reverse the progress of pathological BPH by causing prostate shrinkage and preventing further growth.

**Finasteride** selectively blocks 5α-reductase type 2.

*Efficacy.* Finasteride reduces prostate volume by approximately 20% (Figure 3.2), improving both symptom scores and peak urine flow rate. On average, symptom scores are improved by around one-third after 1 year's treatment, and peak urine flow rate increases by 1.3–1.6 mL/second over 12 months, and possibly more over 4 years (2.3 mL/second in one study). The overall levels of symptoms and quality-of-life impairment associated with BPH are reduced.

The main clinical effects of finasteride may take 3–6 months to become apparent, and patients who benefit most tend to be those with enlarged prostates and serum PSA values > 1.6 ng/mL. The changes in symptom scores and flow rates have been shown to be maintained for at least 5 years. Urodynamic studies have confirmed that prostatic enlargement, flow rates and voiding pressure can be improved significantly by finasteride.

*Adverse effects.* Finasteride is very well tolerated. The main side effects associated with finasteride are reduced libido and erectile dysfunction, each of which occurs in 3–5% of patients. These appear to be reversible on stopping treatment. Some patients may notice a reduction in the volume of ejaculate, and they should be counseled about this. About 1% of men may develop breast tenderness and

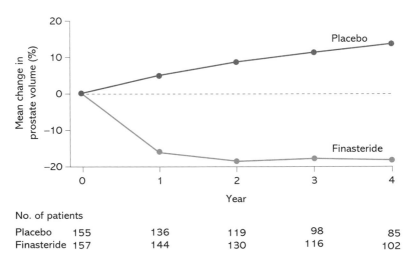

| No. of patients | | | | | |
|---|---|---|---|---|---|
| Placebo | 155 | 136 | 119 | 98 | 85 |
| Finasteride | 157 | 144 | 130 | 116 | 102 |

**Figure 3.2** Treatment with finasteride significantly reduces prostate volume.

some gynecomastia. Women who are or who may potentially be pregnant should not handle crushed or broken tablets. One additional side effect of finasteride, which could be construed as beneficial, is the reduction of male-pattern balding. Patients should be informed of this possibility.

*Outcomes.* Unlike $\alpha_1$-blockers, finasteride appears capable of reversing the natural history of BPH. Figure 3.3 illustrates the reduction in AUR and in the need for surgery in men treated with finasteride in

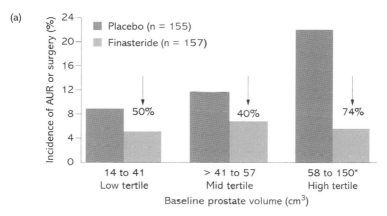

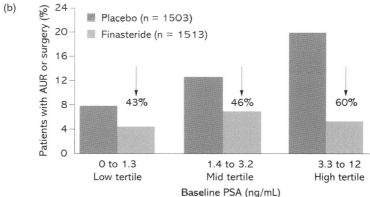

**Figure 3.3** The 4-year incidences of either AUR or surgery related to BPH in patients treated with placebo or finasteride, stratified in tertiles by (a) baseline prostate volume (subset of 10% of patients) or (b) baseline serum prostate-specific antigen (PSA). Arrows denote reduction in risk (log-rank test). *One placebo patient had a prostate volume of 222 cm³.

the 4-year randomized Proscar Long-term Efficacy and Safety Study (PLESS) trial by McConnell et al. The most significant reductions in urinary retention and surgery are seen in men with higher serum PSA levels and larger prostate volumes. Similar responses were seen in the finasteride-alone arm of the MTOPS study (page 49). Serum PSA concentrations are reduced by about 50% after 6–12 months' treatment; thus PSA values in finasteride-treated patients may be multiplied by two and the usual cut-off values still applied. There is no evidence that this reduction in serum PSA limits the value of the test as a cancer detection tool.

**Dutasteride** is a dual 5α-reductase inhibitor.

*Efficacy.* The dual inhibition of types 1 and 2 5α-reductase by dutasteride produces greater suppression of DHT than that achieved with the selective 5α-reductase type 2 inhibitor finasteride. In a 2-year placebo-controlled study, dutasteride significantly improved symptoms and flow. The magnitude of the improvement could be correlated with the prostate volume; men with larger prostates benefited most. Dutasteride also lowers the risk of acute retention and surgery related to BPH by 48–57%.

The results of a pivotal, multicenter trial of dutasteride have recently been published. The drug was shown to reduce the plasma level of DHT by 93%, compared with the 70% reduction achieved with the selective type-2 inhibitor finasteride. In a combined analysis of approximately 4000 patients followed for 4 years, dutasteride was found to achieve an AUA symptom score reduction and maximal flow rate improvement equivalent to finasteride (Figure 3.4). It also reduced the BII to a statistically significant degree compared with placebo. The 52% reduction in serum PSA and 20–25% reduction in prostate volume were also similar to those achieved with finasteride.

*Adverse effects.* The incidence of impotence, decreased libido and ejaculatory disorders is similar to that with finasteride. Gynecomastia and nipple tenderness are seen in 1–1.9% of patients annually.

*Outcomes.* Overall, dutasteride produced a 57% reduction in the risk of AUR and a 48% reduction in the need for BPH-related surgery (Figures 3.5 and 3.6). These overall risk reductions are similar to that

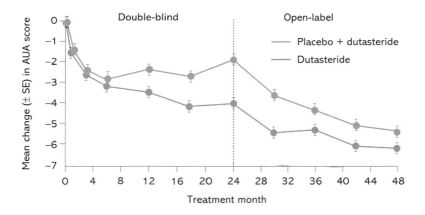

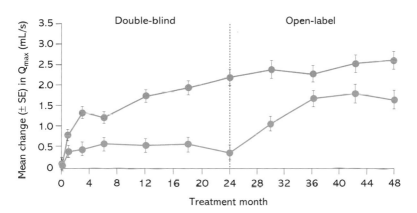

**Figure 3.4** Mean changes in AUA score and maximal flow rate ($Q_{max}$) from baseline over 48 months for dutasteride and placebo treatments. Reproduced from Roehrborn, Marks et al., copyright © 2004, with permission from Elsevier.

seen in the finasteride PLESS trial. Clearly dutasteride is an effective $5\alpha$-reductase inhibitor for the treatment of BPH.

**Impact of $5\alpha$-reductase inhibitors on prostate cancer prevention.** The Prostate Cancer Prevention Trial (PCPT) has raised the possibility that, as well as their action on BPH, $5\alpha$-reductase inhibitors may have some efficacy in prostate cancer prevention. The PCPT reported a statistically significant risk reduction in the prevalence of prostate cancer confirmed by biopsy in patients receiving finasteride over 7 years compared with

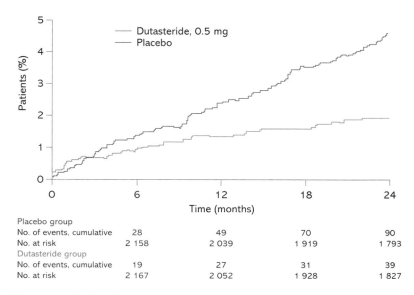

| Placebo group | | | | |
|---|---|---|---|---|
| No. of events, cumulative | 28 | 49 | 70 | 90 |
| No. at risk | 2 158 | 2 039 | 1 919 | 1 793 |
| Dutasteride group | | | | |
| No. of events, cumulative | 19 | 27 | 31 | 39 |
| No. at risk | 2 167 | 2 052 | 1 928 | 1 827 |

**Figure 3.5** Kaplan–Meier curve for first episode of acute urinary retention over 24 months. Reproduced from Roehrborn et al. © 2002, with permission from Elsevier.

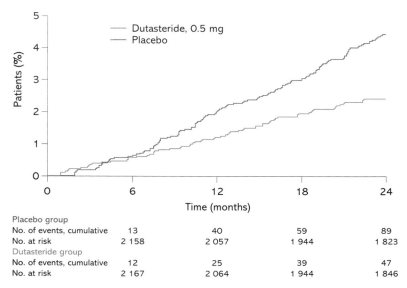

| Placebo group | | | | |
|---|---|---|---|---|
| No. of events, cumulative | 13 | 40 | 59 | 89 |
| No. at risk | 2 158 | 2 057 | 1 944 | 1 823 |
| Dutasteride group | | | | |
| No. of events, cumulative | 12 | 25 | 39 | 47 |
| No. at risk | 2 167 | 2 064 | 1 944 | 1 846 |

**Figure 3.6** Kaplan–Meier curve for first episode of BPH-related surgery over 24 months. Reproduced from Roehrborn et al. © 2002, with permission from Elsevier.

placebo ($p < 0.001$). Patients given finasteride also benefited from a decrease in urinary symptoms and BPH-related events. However, although the incidence of prostate cancer was lower in the finasteride arm, those patients receiving finasteride who did have prostate cancer appeared to have tumors of a higher Gleason grade (7–10). The explanation for this finding is still unclear, but it could conceivably be an artifact, if the Gleason grading system is confounded by the 5$\alpha$-reductase inhibitor effect on gland architecture.

A chemoprevention study with dutasteride, the REDUCE study, is currently under way, since type 1 5$\alpha$-reductase is overexpressed in some prostate cancers, and dutasteride inhibits both isoenzymes. Retrospective analyses of three double-blind, placebo-controlled studies of the efficacy and tolerability of dutasteride in men suffering from BPH revealed that prostate cancer, recorded as an adverse event, was 51% lower in the dutasteride- than in the placebo-treated patients at 27 months (crude incidence rates 1.2% and 2.5%, $p = 0.002$).

**Combination therapy.** As in asthma, where a combination of a bronchodilator (for acute relief) together with a steroid aerosol (to prevent attacks) is employed, combination therapy for BPH with an $\alpha_1$-blocker and a 5$\alpha$-reductase inhibitor appears attractive. Such an approach has been evaluated in several four-arm randomized placebo-controlled studies. The Veterans' Administration Cooperative Study comparing terazosin, finasteride, combination therapy and placebo suggested that the $\alpha_1$-blocker was more effective over 1 year than finasteride, but caused more side effects, particularly dizziness. The mean prostate volume of the men recruited into this study was rather low (36.3 cm$^3$), and it has been suggested that this may have confounded the results. A meta-analysis of almost 5000 patients has revealed, not surprisingly, that finasteride is most effective in men with enlarged prostates (> 30 cm$^3$) and PSA values over 1.4 ng/mL. These effects of prostate volume and PSA were also seen in the PLESS trial (Figure 3.7), but not in the Medical Treatment of Prostatic Symptoms (MTOPS) study.

A four-arm, randomized placebo-controlled study, the PREDICT trial, compared finasteride, doxazosin, a combination of both, and

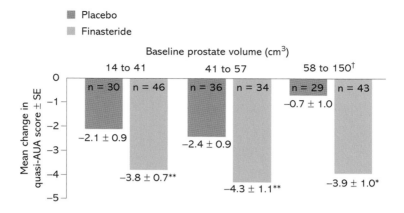

**Figure 3.7** Symptom score responses at year 4 stratified by baseline prostate volume tertiles in men who completed the PLESS study. *$p = < 0.005$; **$p = 0.17$ versus placebo; †only 1 patient had a prostate volume over 150 cm³.

placebo, and essentially reached the same conclusion as the Veterans' Administration investigators.

The five-year, 3000-man MTOPS study demonstrated that the combination of an $\alpha_1$-blocker (doxazosin) and a 5α-reductase inhibitor (finasteride) was more effective than either drug alone in delaying the clinical progression of BPH and improving lower urinary tract symptoms and maximal urinary flow rate (Figure 3.8). Clinical progression in MTOPS was defined as one of the following events: ≥ 4-point increase in AUA symptom score, acute urinary retention (AUR), incontinence, renal insufficiency or recurrent UTI. Doxazosin and finasteride produced equivalent reductions in the risk of progression (39% and 34% reduction, respectively), while combination therapy produced a much more significant 66% reduction in the risk of progression (Figure 3.8). Although doxazosin delayed the short-term risk of AUR and the need for invasive therapy, only finasteride and combination therapy demonstrated significant long-term reduction in these two risks. The MTOPS study clearly demonstrates that, in the long term, combination therapy is more effective than monotherapy in men with LUTS and prostate enlargement – the mean prostate volume in the MTOPS study was 36.3 cm³. Combination therapy was also

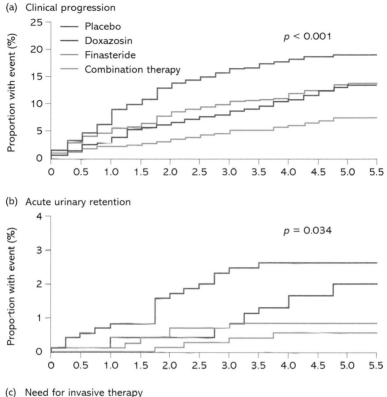

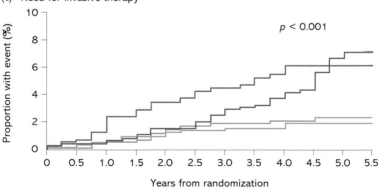

Figure 3.8 Cumulative incidence of: (a) overall BPH progression, (b) acute urinary retention, and (c) crossover to invasive therapy in the four arms of the MTOPS trial. Reproduced with permission from McConnell et al., copyright © 2003 Massachusetts Medical Society. All rights reserved.

shown to be well tolerated by the patients. It can be safely assumed that dutasteride in combination with an α-blocker would be as effective and well-tolerated as any finasteride–α-blocker combination.

A variation on the theme of combination therapy is the use of a 5α-reductase inhibitor in combination with an $\alpha_1$-blocker for 24 weeks, followed by 5α-reductase inhibitor monotherapy. This treatment was found to be effective in the Symptom Management After Reducing Therapy (SMART-1) study, which used dutasteride and tamsulosin as the active agents (Figure 3.9). After cessation of $\alpha_1$-blocker therapy at 24 weeks, dutasteride appeared capable of maintaining the flow rate and symptom improvement.

## Other options

**Phytotherapy.** Various plant extracts have been used to treat BPH in Europe for many years and are becoming increasingly popular in the USA. There are, however, few controlled data to suggest that many of these compounds have anything much other than a placebo effect. In

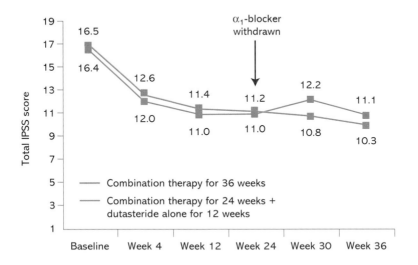

**Figure 3.9.** SMART-1 trial: mean total IPSS for men receiving 36 weeks of combination therapy and for men receiving 24 weeks of combination therapy followed by 5α-reductase inhibitor monotherapy. Reproduced from Barkin et al., copyright © 2003, with permission from the European Association of Urology.

one study, β-sitosterol significantly improved symptom scores and uroflow; another study revealed that a plant extract of *Serenoa repens*, Permixon®, was as effective as finasteride, but unfortunately no placebo arm was utilized in this study. The US National Institutes of Health (NIH) are currently planning a longer-term placebo-controlled study to confirm or refute the safety and efficacy of phytotherapy for BPH.

**Active surveillance.** A strategy of active surveillance is appropriate for patients with very mild BPH symptoms (IPSS ≤ 8) in whom prostate cancer has been excluded, and for more symptomatic patients who are not unduly bothered by their symptoms. Management of such patients involves:

- instruction on appropriate lifestyle changes (e.g. avoiding drinking large volumes in the evening)
- evaluation of symptoms and physical signs, and blood and urine analyses at regular intervals (e.g. annually)
- a PSA test in selected men with a life expectancy of at least 10 years to assess the risk of prostate cancer and BPH progression.

---

**Key points – medical management of BPH**

- α-blockers result in rapid improvement of BPH-related symptoms and urinary flow rate.
- Side effects of α-blockers include tiredness, dizziness and nasal stuffiness.
- 5α-reductase inhibitors shrink the prostate by around 20%.
- This shrinkage improves symptoms, increases flow rate and reduces the rate of BPH progression.
- Side effects of 5α-reductase inhibitors include an incidence of sexual dysfunction of around 3–5%.
- Combination therapy has recently been shown to be the most effective medical means of preventing BPH progression.

---

## Key references

Abrams P, Schulman C, Vaage S and the European Tamsulosin Study Group. Tamsulosin, a selective $\alpha_1$c-adrenoceptor antagonist: a randomized controlled trial in patients with benign prostatic 'obstruction' (symptomatic BPH). *Br J Urol* 1995;76:325–36.

Andersen J, Nickel C, Marshall V et al. Finasteride significantly reduces the occurrence of acute urinary retention and surgical interventions in patients with symptomatic benign prostatic hyperplasia. *Urology* 1997; 49:839–45.

Andriole G, Bostwick D, Brawley O et al. Chemoprevention of prostate cancer in men at high risk: rationale and design of the Reduction by Dutasteride of Prostate Cancer Events (REDUCE) trial. *J Urol* 2004;172: 1314–17.

Andriole GL, Roehrborn C, Schulman C et al. Effect of dutasteride on the detection of prostate cancer in men with benign prostatic hyperplasia. *Urology* 2004; 64:537–41.

Barkin J, Guimaraes M, Jacobi G et al. $\alpha$-blocker therapy can be withdrawn in the majority of men following initial combination therapy with the dual $5\alpha$-reductase inhibitor dutasteride. *Eur Urol* 2003;44:461–6.

Boyle P, Gould A, Roehrborn C. Prostate volume predicts outcome of treatment of benign prostatic hyperplasia with finasteride: meta-analysis of randomised clinical trials. *Urology* 1996;48:398–405.

Boyle P, Siami P, Wachs BH et al. Effect of dutasteride on the risk of acute urinary retention and the need for surgical treatment. *J Urol* 2002; 167:372A.

Buzelin JM, Delauche-Cavallier MC, Roth S et al. Clinical uroselectivity: evidence from patients treated with slow-release alfuzosin for symptomatic benign prostatic obstruction. *Br J Urol* 1997;79: 898–906.

Buzelin JM, Roth S, Geffriaud-Ricouard C, Delauche-Cavallier MC. Efficacy and safety of sustained-release alfuzosin 5 mg in patients with benign prostatic hyperplasia. *Eur Urol* 1997;31:190–8.

Carraro JC, Raynaud JP, Koch G et al. Comparison of phytotherapy (Permixon®) with finasteride in the treatment of benign prostatic hyperplasia: a randomised international study of 1098 patients. *Prostate* 1996;29:231–40.

Clark RV, Hermann DJ, Gabriel H et al. Effective suppression of dihydrotestosterone (DHT) by G1198745, a novel, dual 5-alpha-reductase inhibitor. *J Urol* 1999; 161:268A.

de Mey C, Michel MC, McEwen J, Moreland T. A double blind comparison of terazosin and tamsulosin on their differential effects on ambulatory blood pressure and nocturnal orthostatic stress testing. *Eur Urol* 1998;33:481–8.

Fabricius PG, Weizert P, Dunzendorfer U et al. Efficacy of once-a-day terazosin in benign prostatic hyperplasia: A randomized placebo controlled clinical trial. *Prostate* 1990;(suppl 3):85–93.

Finasteride Study Group. Finasteride (MK906) in the treatment of benign prostatic hyperplasia. *Prostate* 1993; 22:291–9.

Gormley GJ, Stoner E, Bruskewitz RC et al. The effect of finasteride in men with benign prostatic hyperplasia. *N Engl J Med* 1992;327: 1185–91.

Kawabe K, Niijina T. Use of an alpha1-blocker, YM12617, in micturition difficulty. *Urol Int* 1987;42:280–4.

Kirby RS. Doxazosin in benign prostatic hyperplasia: effects on blood pressure and urinary flow in normotensive and hypertensive men. *Urology* 1995;46(2):182–6.

Kirby RS. Profile of doxazosin in hypertensive men with benign prostatic hyperplasia. *Br J Clin Pract* 1994;54 (suppl):23–8.

Kirby RS, Coppinger SWC, Corcoran MO et al. Prazosin in the treatment of prostatic obstruction. A placebo controlled study. *Br J Urol* 1987;60:136–42.

Kirby RS, Pool JL. Alpha-adrenoceptor blockade in the treatment of benign prostatic hyperplasia: past, present and future. *Br J Urol* 1997;80:521–32.

Kirby RS, Roehrborn C, Boyle P et al. Efficacy and tolerability of doxazosin and finasteride, alone or in combination, in treatment of symptomatic benign prostatic hyperplasia: the Prospective European Doxazosin and Combination Therapy (PREDICT) trial. *Urology* 2003;61:119–26.

Lepor H, Auerbach S, PurasBaez A et al. A randomised, placebo-controlled multicentre study of the efficacy and safety of terazosin in the treatment of benign prostatic hyperplasia. *J Urol* 1992;148: 1467–74.

Lepor H, Williford WO, Barry MJ et al. The efficacy of terazosin, finasteride or both in benign prostatic hypertrophy. *N Engl J Med* 1996; 335:533–9.

McConnell JD, Bruskewitz R, Walsh PC et al. The effect of finasteride on the risk of acute urinary retention and the need for surgical treatment among men with benign prostatic hyperplasia. Finasteride Long-Term Efficacy and Safety Study Group. *N Engl J Med* 1998;338:557–63.

McConnell JD and the PLESS Study Group. The long-term effects of finasteride on BPH: results of a four-year, placebo-controlled study. *Br J Urol* 1997;80(suppl 2):182.

McConnell JD, Roehrborn CG, Bautista OM et al. The long-term effect of doxazosin, finasteride, and combination therapy on the clinical progression of benign prostatic hyperplasia. *N Engl J Med* 2003; 349:2387–98.

McNeill SA. The role of alpha-blockers in the management of acute urinary retention caused by benign prostatic obstruction. *Eur Urol* 2004;45:325–32.

O'Leary MP, Roehrborn C, Andriole G et al. Improvements in benign prostatic hyperplasia-specific quality of life with dutasteride, the novel dual 5alpha-reductase inhibitor. *BJU Int* 2003;92:262–6.

Roehrborn C, Boyle P, Nickel J et al. ARIA3001 ARIA3002 and ARIA3003 Study Investigators. Efficacy and safety of a dual inhibitor of 5-alpha-reductase types 1 and 2 (dutasteride) in men with benign prostatic hyperplasia. *Urology* 2002;60:434–41.

Roehrborn CG, Marks LS, Fenter T et al. Efficacy and safety of dutasteride in the four-year treatment of men with benign prostatic hyperplasia. *Urology* 2004;63: 709–15.

Roehrborn CG, Ramsdell J, Siami P. Prostate volume at baseline predicts the margin of therapeutic response with the 5$\alpha$-reductase inhibitor dutasteride. *J Urol* 2002;167:373A.

Roehrborn CG, Schwinn DA. Alpha1-adrenergic receptors and their inhibitors in lower urinary tract symptoms and benign prostatic hyperplasia. *J Urol* 2004;171: 1029–35.

Speakman MJ, Kirby RS, Joyce A et al. Guideline for the primary care management of male lower urinary tract symptoms. *BJU Int* 2004;93: 985–90.

Stoner E. Three-year safety and efficacy data on the use of finasteride in the treatment of benign prostatic hyperplasia. *Urology* 1994;43:284–9.

Thompson IM, Goodman PJ, Tangen CM et al. The influence of finasteride on the development of prostate cancer. *N Engl J Med* 2003;349: 215–24.

Surgical treatment is usually indicated for patients who have complications of BPH and for those who have symptoms that are inadequately controlled by medical therapy or who elect to forego a trial of medical therapy and to receive more definitive treatment (Table 4.1). Three standard options are available:
- transurethral resection of the prostate (TURP)
- transurethral incision of the prostate (TUIP)
- open prostatectomy.

In general, surgical treatment produces the best improvements in symptoms and urine flow rates, and has a lower requirement for further therapy but a higher incidence of complications than medical treatment (Table 4.2).

## Transurethral resection of the prostate

About 95% of prostatectomies are still carried out by TURP. A resectoscope with a diathermy loop is introduced via the urethra, and chips of hyperplastic tissue are excised and removed through the resectoscope sheath (Figure 4.1). The operation can be performed under spinal epidural or light general anesthesia; a urethral catheter is retained

---

TABLE 4.1

**Indications for prostatectomy in patients with BPH**

- Acute urinary retention
- Chronic urinary retention due to prostatic obstruction
- Recurrent urinary tract infections/hematuria
- Bladder stones secondary to BPH
- Renal insufficiency due to BPH
- Large bladder diverticulum/diverticula
- Bothersome LUTS persisting after medical therapy
- Patient preference

TABLE 4.2

Outcome and complications of transurethral resection of the prostate (TURP), transurethral incision of the prostate (TUIP) and open prostatectomy

| | TURP | TUIP | Open prostatectomy |
|---|---|---|---|
| **Outcome** | | | |
| Likelihood of symptom improvement (%) | 90 | 80 | 98 |
| Reduction in symptom score (%) | 85 | 73 | 79 |
| Improvement in mean peak flow rate (mL/s) | 8–18 | 8–15 | 8–23 |
| Likelihood of further surgery within 8 years (%) | 16–20 | > 20 | 10 |
| **Complications** | | | |
| Overall rate (%) | 16.1 | 14 | 21.7 |
| Risk of blood transfusion (%) | < 15 | 2 | < 30 |
| Incontinence (%) | 0.2–1 | < 0.1 | 0.4 |
| Erectile dysfunction (%) | 2–5 | < 2 | 19 |
| Retrograde ejaculation (%) | 70–90 | 10 | 72 |
| Need for operative treatment of surgical complications (%) | 3.3 | 2.9 | 4.2 |
| Likelihood of death within 90 days of surgery (%) | 0.2–1.5 | < 1 | 2 |

for 36–48 hours postoperatively. Symptoms are improved in about 70–90% of patients, and peak urine flow rates of well over 15–20 mL/second can be achieved reliably.

**Complications.** Although postoperative erectile dysfunction has been reported in a proportion (2–5%) of men undergoing TURP, there is no clear rationale for this, and it is probable that many cases may be psychosomatic or simply the result of aging. Indeed, postoperative

(a)  (b)

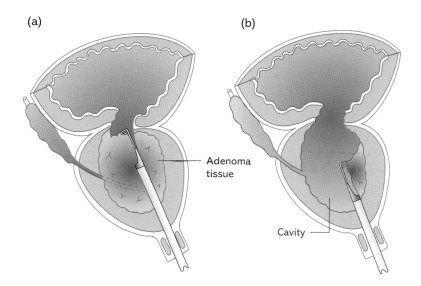

Adenoma tissue

Cavity

**Figure 4.1** In transurethral resection of the prostate, (a) the median lobe is resected and (b) lateral adenoma tissue removed, leaving a cavity that subsequently epithelializes over 4–6 weeks.

impotence has been reported in about 4% of men undergoing general surgical procedures not involving the genitourinary tract. Other studies suggest that erectile dysfunction following TURP is no more common than in a similar group of men managed by active surveillance. One study even provided evidence that sexual function actually improved after TURP.

Retrograde ejaculation is the most common sequela of TURP (Table 4.2 and Figure 4.2). It results from loss of the bladder-neck sphincter mechanism; the bladder neck does not close during ejaculation, and semen passes retrogradely into the bladder rather than through the urethra. Patients who have been adequately informed preoperatively about the possibility of retrograde ejaculation do not usually find it too troublesome, but it is irreversible.

Other complications of TURP include perioperative and secondary hemorrhage (anticoagulants, antiplatelet medications and aspirin should be stopped preoperatively), incontinence due to sphincter injury (< 1%) and urethral stricture (Table 4.2). Although incontinence is very

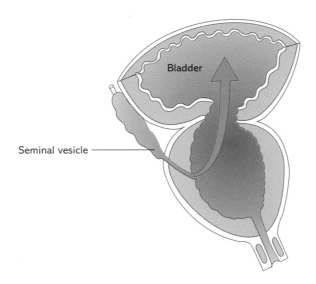

**Figure 4.2** Retrograde ejaculation, resulting from loss of the bladder-neck sphincter mechanism, is a common sequela of TURP.

uncommon after TURP, when it does occur, it is associated with a profound reduction in quality of life. Most patients also complain of dysuria and urgency of micturition for several weeks after surgery. If this symptom persists, urinary tract infection should be excluded. Nowadays less than 5% of patients undergoing TURP will require a blood transfusion; occasionally a urethral stricture may develop. This requires further intervention, but usually responds to treatment.

**Outcomes.** TURP and open prostatectomy provide greater improvements in symptoms and urine flow rates than any other BPH treatment currently available except, perhaps, holmium laser prostatectomy. However, although most patients are satisfied with the outcome after TURP, 10–20% may have a less than perfect result. This may reflect inappropriate patient selection. Careful evaluation of the impact of symptoms on everyday life and scrupulous identification of the presence and severity of obstruction can help to optimize the outcome after TURP. Where patients are properly selected and the surgeon is skillful, the morbidity rate should be less than 10%, and mortality should be considerably less than 1%.

In the longer term, prostatic regrowth or other problems may necessitate a further TURP. Overall, a reoperation rate of 20% over 8 years of follow-up has been reported.

## Transurethral incision of the prostate

TUIP may be the procedure of choice in patients with a prostate that, although relatively small, still causes obstruction. It is suitable only for smaller prostates (≤ 30 g resectable tissue) with a high bladder neck and no middle-lobe hyperplasia. The procedure involves making an incision through the bladder neck from just below the ureteric orifice to a point about 0.1 cm proximal to the verumontanum (Figure 4.3). TUIP is almost as effective as TURP in relieving symptoms, and may produce similar increases in urine flow rates. Incidence of complications, such as bleeding, stricture or incontinence, is lower than that of TURP; in

(a)

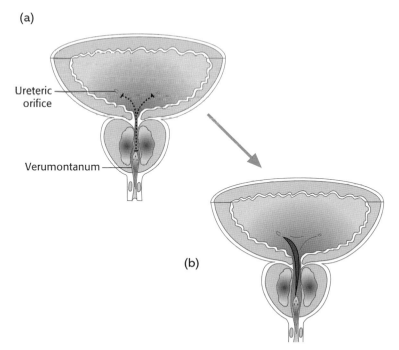

Ureteric orifice

Verumontanum

(b)

**Figure 4.3** Transurethral incision of the prostate: (a) An incision is made through the bladder neck (dotted lines) to separate the two lateral lobes. (b) The incision is usually unilateral, but may be bilateral.

---

**Key points – surgical management of BPH**

- TURP is the chosen method of surgery in 95% of cases.
- Indications for surgery include complications of BPH or failure to respond to medical treatment.
- Outcomes in terms of flow rate and symptom reduction are usually good.
- Complications such as bleeding or clot retention occur in around 16% of cases.
- Retrograde ejaculation is usual but seldom troublesome.
- Open prostatectomy is confined to those with glands of volume > 100 $cm^3$.

---

particular, retrograde ejaculation is markedly less common, occurring in only about 10% of patients. The likelihood that further treatment will eventually be necessary, however, may be somewhat higher after TUIP than after TURP (Table 4.2).

## Open prostatectomy

Open prostatectomy is now indicated only for individuals with a very large prostate and those who have coexistent pathology such as a sizeable bladder stone. Open prostatectomy is performed through a midline or transverse suprapubic incision in the lower abdomen. Two approaches are used:

- retropubic prostatectomy (Millin's prostatectomy), in which the prostatic capsule is incised and the adenoma enucleated by the urologist's finger (Figure 4.4)
- transvesical (suprapubic) prostatectomy, in which access to the prostate is gained via an incision in the bladder.

Open prostatectomy improves symptoms in most patients (Table 4.2), and peak urine flow rate usually increases to over 20 mL/second. Moreover, the need for a further operation is considerably lower among patients undergoing open prostatectomy than those undergoing TURP. Because the procedure is invasive, however, patients require a longer stay in hospital than after TURP,

(a)

(b)

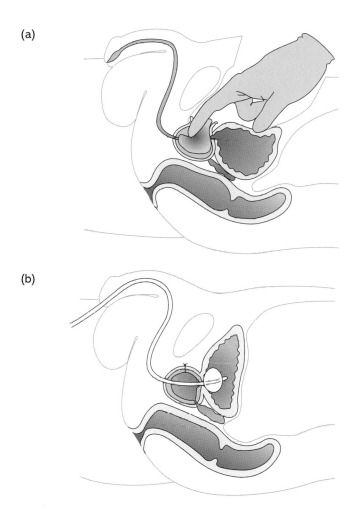

**Figure 4.4** (a) In an open prostatectomy the hyperplastic tissue is enucleated via an incision in the prostatic capsule (as here) or bladder. (b) A urethral catheter is then inserted and left in situ for 3–5 days.

and postoperative complications are more common (Table 4.2). Thus, most surgeons now opt for TURP, except for patients with the very largest of glands (> 100 cm$^3$).

## Key references

Abrams PH, Farrar DJ, Turner Warwick RT et al. The results of prostatectomy: a symptomatic and urodynamic analysis of 152 patients. *J Urol* 1979;121:640–2.

Bruskewitz RC, Larsen EH, Madsen PO, Dorflinger T. 3-year follow-up of urinary symptoms after transurethral resection of the prostate. *J Urol* 1986;136:613–15.

Emberton M, Black N, Blandy JP et al. The effectiveness of prostatectomy in reducing symptoms and improving quality of life in 5131 men. *J Urol* 1995;153:317A.

Holtgrewe HL, Valk WL. Factors influencing mortality and morbidity of transurethral prostatectomy: a study of 2013. *J Urol* 1962;87: 450–549.

Larsen EH, Dorflinger T, Gasser TC et al. Transurethral incision versus transurethral resection of the prostate for the treatment of benign prostatic hypertrophy. A preliminary report. *Scand J Urol Nephrol* 1987;104: 83–6.

Mebust WK, Holtgrewe HL, Cockett ATK. Transurethral prostatectomy: immediate and postoperative complications: a cooperative study of 13 participating institutions evaluating 3885 patients. *J Urol* 1989;141:243–7.

Roos NP, Ramsey EW. A population based study of prostatectomy: outcomes associated with differing surgical approaches. *J Urol* 1987; 137:1184–8.

Roos NP, Wennberg JE, Malenka DJ et al. Mortality and reoperation after open and transurethral resection of the prostate for benign prostatic hyperplasia. *N Engl J Med* 1989; 320:1120–4.

Wasson JH, Reda DJ, Bruskewitz RC et al. A comparison of transurethral surgery with watchful waiting for moderate symptoms of benign prostatic hyperplasia. *N Engl J Med* 1995;332:75–9.

A number of minimally invasive techniques for the treatment of BPH have been developed and evaluated in recent years (Table 5.1). Most are designed to reduce the volume of the transition zone and thereby relieve the 'static' component of obstruction. As yet, however, none of these new approaches has been shown to equal the consistent long-term improvements in symptoms and urine flow rates and the low reoperation rate achieved with TURP. Most of these techniques should still be regarded as investigational, but they are nonethless often eagerly requested by patients.

## Prostatic stents

Temporary or permanent stents have been used to maintain expansion of the prostatic urethra. Although they are effective in relieving obstruction in patients with urinary retention, they provide only modest improvements in symptom scores and urine flow rates in patients with BPH without retention. Stents are also subject to complications, such as encrustation with calcium salts and obstructive growth of prostatic epithelium through the mesh, and may cause

TABLE 5.1

Minimally invasive approaches for BPH

- Prostatic stents
- Electrovaporization
- Laser ablation
    - endoscopic laser ablation of the prostate
    - interstitial laser therapy
    - holmium laser resection
- Transurethral needle ablation (TUNA)
- Transurethral microwave thermotherapy (TUMT)

prolonged urethral discomfort and irritation. As a result, their use is currently restricted to those very few patients with outflow obstruction who are unsuitable for conventional surgical procedures.

## Electrovaporization

A modification of the standard TURP instrument, the VaporTrode™ (Figure 5.1), permits vaporization of prostate tissue with a grooved 'roller-ball' electrode that creates zones of high current density. A number of studies show an outcome similar to TURP, with less hemorrhage, but long-term outcome data are still needed.

## Laser ablation

Laser ablation with the neodymium–YAG laser has been evaluated in a number of centers. Several approaches have been used:

- endoscopic laser ablation of the prostate (ELAP), in which a side-firing probe is inserted via a cystoscope (Figure 5.2)
- interstitial laser, in which the lateral lobes are perforated with a laser fiber and laser energy is applied to the interior of the adenoma.

Recent studies with the latter technique have reported a greater than 50% improvement in symptom scores as well as an increase in peak urine flow rate of 3–6 mL/second. As with electrovaporization, blood loss is minimal. Some patients may, however, experience postoperative pain and difficulty in passing urine for some weeks, because laser ablation involves higher temperatures than either hyperthermia or thermotherapy. For this reason, suprapubic catheterization may be necessary for several days or even weeks after the procedure, increasing

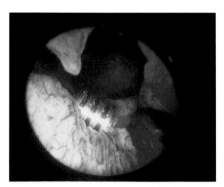

**Figure 5.1** The VaporTrode™.

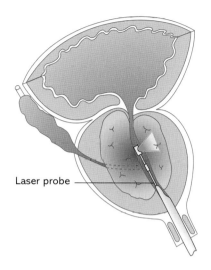

**Figure 5.2** In endoscopic laser ablation of the prostate, a side-firing probe is inserted through a cystoscope, and laser energy is applied to the affected area under direct vision.

Laser probe

the likelihood of urinary tract infection. Large-scale comparisons with TURP to compare the long-term benefits and risks of laser ablation with conventional surgery suggest that TURP is more effective, especially in terms of avoiding secondary, unplanned catheterization, although less bleeding occurs with laser ablation.

The development of interstitial laser therapy, whereby a laser fiber is introduced into the center of the benignly enlarged prostate, is currently under investigation (Figure 5.3). Early results seem encouraging in

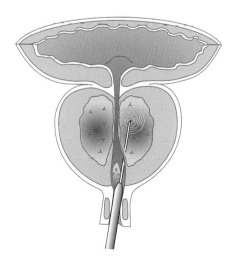

**Figure 5.3** In interstitial laser therapy, a fiber is used to perforate the adenoma. Energy is applied to the center of the adenoma, thereby preserving the urethral epithelium but reducing adenoma bulk.

terms of efficacy and side effects, perhaps because the urethra is spared by these devices, but long-term randomized outcome evaluations are still awaited.

Unlike the Nd–YAG laser, the holmium laser permits actual tissue resection (Figure 5.4). In this respect it is equivalent to TURP, but it causes less bleeding, and TURP syndrome is absent. The holmium laser has been used for enucleation of very large glands and subsequent intravesical tissue morcellation. In the hands of an experienced surgeon, the technique has results comparable to or better than those of open prostatectomy, especially in terms of blood loss. The tissue morcellator must be used with caution, however, because of the risk of perforating or injuring the bladder wall.

## Transurethral needle ablation

Transurethral needle ablation (TUNA) uses radiofrequency energy to apply high temperatures (120°C) to the prostate with minimal damage to the prostatic urethra (Figure 5.5). Increases in peak urine flow rates comparable to those achieved with TURP (9–17 mL/second) have been reported by some investigators. Unlike most other minimally invasive

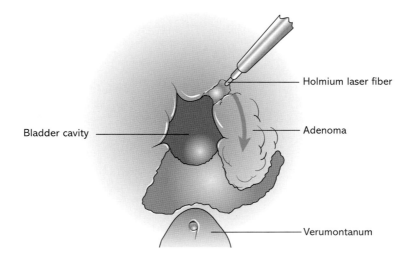

Bladder cavity

Holmium laser fiber

Adenoma

Verumontanum

**Figure 5.4** Holmium laser resection of the prostate.

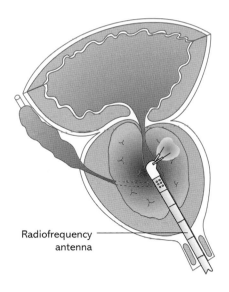

**Figure 5.5** Transurethral needle ablation uses a radiofrequency antenna to raise the temperature of the center of the enlarged prostate to 120°C without damaging the prostatic urethra.

Radiofrequency antenna

techniques, this approach requires only local anesthetic, and bleeding is minimal, but a relatively long period of catheterization is often necessary. Long-term randomized outcome data suggest that the improvement created is less dramatic than in the case of TURP, but more than can be achieved with medical therapy.

## Transurethral microwave thermotherapy

Transurethral microwave thermotherapy (TUMT) uses a urethral microwave device (Figure 5.6) to heat the prostate to 45–55°C. Damage to the urethra is reputedly prevented by a conductive cooling system. The Prostatron™ unit is the most extensively evaluated device, although other units, such as the Targis™ machine, are gaining in popularity, especially in the USA. TUMT has been reported to produce significant improvements in symptom scores and urine flow rates, possibly by inducing tissue necrosis and damaging both intraprostatic nerves and $\alpha_1$-receptors. On average, peak urine flow rate increases by about 2.8–5.3 mL/second (see Table 6.2, page 75). Thus, the effect of TUMT is comparable to that of medical therapy. However, a significant number of patients experience temporary urinary retention after treatment, although this usually resolves with time. New protocols using higher intraprostatic temperatures seem to be producing enhanced

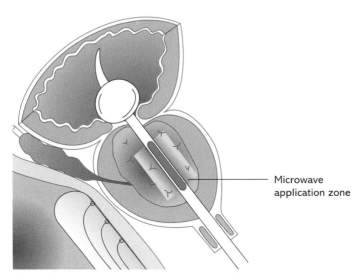

Microwave
application zone

**Figure 5.6** In transurethral microwave thermotherapy, microwave radiation is applied to the prostate by a urethral catheter. Local temperature is monitored by a probe positioned in the rectum, and the urethra is cooled during the procedure.

results, and a proportion of patients prefer the one-off nature of this therapy, which may have less impact on ejaculatory function than TURP, to the chronicity of pharmacotherapy.

---

**Key points – minimally invasive treatment options**

- Prostatic stents can restore voiding in patients with AUR who are unfit for TURP.
- Laser prostatectomy with a holmium laser can remove tissue almost bloodlessly.
- Thermotherapy produces results similar to those achieved by medical therapy in a single treatment.

---

## Key references

d'Ancona FCH, Francisca EAE, Hendriks JCM et al. High energy transurethral thermotherapy in the treatment of benign prostatic hyperplasia: criteria to predict outcome. *Prost Cancer Prost Dis* 1999; 2:98–105.

De La Rosette J, Wildt M, Hofner K et al. High energy thermotherapy in the treatment of benign prostatic hyperplasia: results of the European benign prostatic hyperplasia study group. *J Urol* 1996;156:97–102.

Donatucci C, Donohue R, Berger N et al. Randomized clinical trial comparing balloon dilatation to transurethral resection of prostate for benign prostatic hyperplasia. *Urology* 1993;42:42–9.

Gilling P, Westenberg A, Kennett K et al. Holmium laser resection of the prostate versus transurethral resection of the prostate: results of a randomized trial with 4-year minimum long-term followup. *J Urol* 2004;172:616–19.

Hoffman RM, Macdonald R, Slaton JW et al. Laser prostatectomy versus transurethral resection for treating benign prostatic obstruction: a systematic review. *J Urol* 2003; 169:210–15.

Issa MM. Transurethral needle ablation of the prostate: report of initial United States clinical trial. *J Urol* 1996;156:413–19.

Kaplan SA, Blute M, Bruskewitz RC et al. Long-term efficacy and durability in 345 patients treated with transurethral microwave thermotherapy for benign prostatic hyperplasia: five-year results. *J Urol* 2001;167:292A.

Kuo RL, Kim SC, Lingeman JE et al. Holmium laser enucleation of prostate (HoLEP): the Methodist Hospital experience with greater than 75 gram enucleations. *J Urol* 2003;170:149–52.

Lepor H, Sypherd D, Machi G, Derus J. Randomized double blind study comparing the effectiveness of balloon dilatation of the prostate and cystoscopy for the treatment of symptomatic benign prostatic hyperplasia. *J Urol* 1992;147: 639–44.

McAllister WJ, Karim O, Plail RO et al. Transurethral electrovaporization of the prostate: is it any better than conventional transurethral resection of the prostate? *BJU Int* 2003;91: 211–4.

Rosario D, Woo H, Byrne L et al. 12-month follow-up of the safety and efficacy of TransUrethral Needle Ablation (TUNA). *J Urol* 1996; 155:705A.

Tewari A, Narayan P. Electrovaporisation of the prostate. *Br J Urol* 1996;78:667–76.

Yang Q, Peters TJ, Donovan JL et al. Transurethral incision compared with transurethral resection of the prostate for bladder outlet obstruction: a systematic review and meta-analysis of randomized controlled trials. *J Urol* 2001;165:1526–32.

Zlotta AR, Giannakopoulos X, Maehlum O et al. Long-term evaluation of transurethral needle ablation of the prostate (TUNA) for treatment of symptomatic benign prostatic hyperplasia: clinical outcome up to five years from three centers. *Eur Urol* 2003;44:89–93.

## 6  Considerations in treatment decisions

The choice of treatment for an individual patient with BPH will depend
on a number of factors, including:
- the severity of symptoms, and the extent to which they adversely
  affect the patient's everyday life (i.e. 'bothersomeness')
- the risk of BPH progression
- the long-term efficacy and retreatment rate of therapy
- the likelihood of treatment-associated morbidity or complications
- patient preference
- cost-effectiveness.

### The 'balance-sheet' concept

The most effective treatments are often associated with the
greatest risk of complications. Thus, it is important that the relative
benefits and risks of each treatment option are fully and lucidly
explained to the patient – the 'balance-sheet' concept may be useful
in this context. The AUA's 2003 guideline on the management of
BPH contains detailed, evidence-based comparisons of the outcomes
and adverse effects of both medical and surgical treatments
(Tables 6.1–6.6).

It may also be useful to explain the benefits of treatment in terms
of direct and indirect outcomes. The direct outcome is improvement
in symptoms resulting from treatment; it is this measure which is most
important to the patient. Indirect outcomes, such as improvements in
peak urine flow rate and PVR volume of urine, may be objective and
easy to measure, but are usually less important to the patient. Some
patients, therefore, may be prepared to forego the superior efficacy of
surgical procedures in favor of the lower morbidity associated with
medical therapy, provided their symptoms improve sufficiently. Other
patients may prefer active surveillance even though they have
significant symptoms, because either they are not bothered by them
or they consider the risks of therapy (even medical) to outweigh the
benefit of symptom improvement.

TABLE 6.1

Outcomes of medical therapies: estimates of change in outcome measures after 10–16 months

| | IPSS | $Q_{max}$ (mL/s) | QoL |
|---|---|---|---|
| **α-blockers** | | | |
| Alfuzosin | −4.44* | 2.05* | −1.10* |
| Doxazosin | −5.63 | 2.98 | −1.47 |
| Tamsulosin | −7.53[†] | 1.86[†] | − |
| Terazosin | −5.99 | 1.94 | −1.37 |
| **5α-reductase inhibitors** | | | |
| Finasteride | −3.40 | 1.66 | −0.87 |
| Dutasteride | −3.8 | 1.7 | −0.93 (BII) |
| **Combinations** | | | |
| Alfuzosin/finasteride | − | − | − |
| Doxazosin/finasteride | −6.53 | 3.38 | −1.57 |
| Terazosin/finasteride | −6.21[†] | 2.63 | − |
| Placebo | −2.33[†] | 4.48[†] | −0.67[†] |

*Change in outcome measures over 3–9 months rather than 10–16.

[†]These numbers are based on single-arm analyses – no data available from randomized, controlled trials. Numbers without asterisks are from randomized trials with placebo controls.

Adapted with permission from the American Urological Association 2003, except dutasteride data, from 12-month data in Roehrborn et al. 2002.

BII, BPH impact index; IPSS, International Prostate Symptom Score; $Q_{max}$, peak flow rate; QoL, quality of life score.

As our understanding of the risk factors for progression (large prostate, raised PSA, severe symptoms, increased post-void residual urine and a flow rate < 10 mL/second) has improved, so has our ability to advise BPH sufferers what the future is likely to hold for them with or without therapeutic intervention. The paramount consideration is the effect of BPH on the patient's quality of life (Table 6.7, page 80) and the ability of a given therapy to improve it in the long term versus the risk of any adverse effects.

## Patient preference

The preference of the informed patient, as well as that of his immediate family, is always an important factor in the choice of treatment. Many

TABLE 6.2

**Outcomes of minimally invasive therapies: estimates of change in outcome measures after 10–16 months**

|  | IPSS | $Q_{max}$ (mL/s) | QoL |
|---|---|---|---|
| UroLume stent | −12.44* | 7.80* | – |
| **Thermal-based therapies** | | | |
| Prostatron version 2.0 TUMT | −10.47* | 2.81* | −1.75* |
| Prostatron version 2.5 TUMT | −10.72* | 4.54* | – |
| Targis TUMT | −9.44 | 5.29 | −2.44 |
| TUNA | −9.32 | 4.29 | −2.70 |
| Active surveillance | −0.50* | – | – |
| Sham (control) | – | – | – |
| TURP (control) | −14.80* | 10.77* | −3.34* |

*These numbers are based on single-arm analyses – no data available from randomized, controlled trials. Note that single-arm analyses are the same for TURP comparison. Numbers without asterisks are randomized controlled comparisons to TURP.

Adapted with permission from the American Urological Association 2003.

IPSS, International Prostate Symptom Score; $Q_{max}$, peak flow rate; QoL, quality of life score; TUMT, transurethral microwave thermotherapy; TUNA, transurethral needle ablation; TURP, transurethral resection of the prostate.

patients with mild symptoms opt for active surveillance. Patients with moderate symptoms show a variety of preferences, depending on how bothered they are by their symptoms, and their willingness to accept particular risks (e.g. the risk of retrograde ejaculation); some patients with moderate but bothersome symptoms will be prepared to accept the risks of surgery because of the greater potential benefits and the advantages of a 'once and for all' solution. Patients with severe symptoms are most likely to prefer surgery, but a significant number of these men still choose active surveillance (watchful waiting) or medical treatment. In general, of course, the more severe the symptoms, the more likely is the chance of BPH progression and the greater the chance that the patient will benefit from more invasive therapy such as TURP.

Of the complications that can occur after prostatic surgery, some are more serious than others. A UK study suggested that the induction of retrograde ejaculation by TURP in fact had little or no impact on

TABLE 6.3

Outcomes of surgical therapies: estimates of change in outcome measures after 10–16 months

| | IPSS | $Q_{max}$ (mL/s) | QoL |
|---|---|---|---|
| TURP | −14.80* | 10.77* | −3.34* |
| Holmium laser resection | −17.90* | 10.96* | − |
| Transurethral laser coagulation | −20.20 | 10.97 | − |
| Transurethral incision (TUIP) | −15.19 | 7.65† | −3.67* |
| Transurethral electrovaporization | −15.75* | 12.52* | −3.70* |
| Transurethral laser vaporization | −14.10* | 11.10* | −1.70* |
| Open prostatectomy | − | 11.50* | − |
| Active surveillance | −0.50* | − | − |

*These numbers are based on single-arm analyses – no data available from randomized, controlled trials. †Single-arm numbers used here because the results from randomized, controlled trials were deemed unreasonable. Due most likely to tecnhnique, patient selection or other problems. Numbers without asterisks are based on results from randomized trials with TURP controls.

Adapted with permission from the American Urological Association 2003.

IPSS, International Prostate Symptom Score; $Q_{max}$, peak flow rate; QoL, quality of life score; TURP, transurethral resection of the prostate.

quality of life; in contrast, urinary incontinence or recurrent stricture after TURP had a severely deleterious effect in this respect.

**Unwillingness to seek medical attention.** Although BPH symptoms can have a marked effect on the patient's quality of life, a significant number of men with LUTS resulting from BPH do not seek medical attention (Table 6.8, page 81). Possible reasons for this include embarrassment, a belief that their symptoms are simply a result of aging and thus cannot be treated, or a fear that cancer might be diagnosed. Improved public health education should help to remedy this situation. Primary care physicians also need to be more adequately informed and aware, so that they can correctly identify and initiate treatment in those individuals whose quality of life is affected by this very prevalent disorder of men beyond middle age.

TABLE 6.4

Outcomes of medical therapies: estimates of median percentage rates of adverse events (95% confidence interval)

| | Acute urinary retention | Asthenia | Cardio-vascular | Dizziness | Headache | Hypotension asymptomatic | Sexual: ejaculation | Sexual: erectile problems |
|---|---|---|---|---|---|---|---|---|
| **α-blockers** | | | | | | | | |
| Alfuzosin | – | 4% (1–10) | 1% (0–4) | 5% (1–12) | 5% (3–9) | – | – | 3% (1–6) |
| Doxazosin | 0% (0–1) | 15% (13–18) | 2% (1–4) | 13% (9–19) | 8% (4–12) | 5% (3–10) | 0% (0–2) | 4% (1–8) |
| Tamsulosin | 4% (1–8) | 7% (3–12) | 8% (2–18) | 12% (8–17) | 12% (6–19) | 7% (2–15) | 10% (6–15) | 4% (1–8) |
| Terazosin | 4% (1–8) | 12% (10–13) | 2% (1–3) | 15% (12–20) | 7% (5–10) | 8% (2–18) | 1% (1–2) | 5% (3–8) |
| **5α-reductase inhibitors** | | | | | | | | |
| Finasteride | * | – | – | – | – | – | 4% (3–5) | 8% (6–11) |
| Dutasteride | * | – | – | – | – | – | 2.2% | 7.3% |
| **Combinations** | | | | | | | | |
| Alfuzosin/ finasteride | 0% (0–1) | 1% (0–2) | – | 2% (1–4) | 2% (1–3) | 8% (6–11) | 1% (0–2) | 8% (5–11) |
| Doxazosin/ finasteride | 0% (0–1) | 13% (9–17) | 2% (1–4) | 14% (11–19) | 9% (6–13) | 3% (1–5) | 3% (2–6) | 10% (7–14) |
| Terazosin/ finasteride | – | 14% (11–18) | – | 21% (17–26) | 5% (3–8) | – | 7% (5–10) | 9% (1–13) |
| Placebo | 3% (2–5) | 4% (3–5) | 4% (2–7) | 5% (4–7) | 5% (4–7) | 2% (1–3) | 1% (1–1) | 4% (3–5) |

Adapted with permission from the American Urological Association BPH Guidelines 2003, except for dutasteride data, published by Roehrborn et al. 2002 (confidence intervals not available). *Reduced the risk of acute urinary retention by 57% compared with placebo (McConnell et al. 1998; Roehrborn et al. 2002).

TABLE 6.5

## Outcomes of minimally invasive therapies: estimates of median percentage rates of adverse events (95% confidence interval)

| | Aborted procedure/ device failure | Acute urinary retention | Incontinence | Infection/ UTI | Sexual: ejaculation | Sexual: erectile problems | Transfusion |
|---|---|---|---|---|---|---|---|
| UroLume stent | 34% (11–64) | 6% (2–15) | 25% (7–53) | 11% (6–18) | – | – | – |
| **Thermal-based therapies** | | | | | | | |
| Prostatron version 2.0 TUMT | 1% (0–3) | 23% (18–29) | 2% (1–4) | 9% (5–15) | 5% (4–8) | 3% (1–5) | 1% (0–4) |
| Prostatron version 2.5 TUMT | – | 15% (4–33) | – | 9% (3–19) | 16% (2–49) | 1% (0–8) | 2% (0–9) |
| Targis TUMT | 1% (0–4) | 6% (1–17) | – | 9% (5–15) | 5% (2–10) | – | 0% (0–2) |
| TUNA | 4% (1–9) | 20% (13–29) | 1% (0–4) | 17% (9–29) | 4% (1–10) | 3% (1–6) | 3% (1–8) |
| Active surveillance | – | 3% (2–6) | 2% (1–3) | 0% (0–1) | – | 21% (17–26) | 0% (0–1) |
| Sham (control) | 1% (0–6) | 3% (1–5) | 1% (0–6) | 5% (2–11) | 2% (0–5) | 2% (1–6) | 1% (0–6) |
| TURP (control) | – | 3% (4–8) | 3% (2–5) | 6% (5–9) | 65% (56–72) | 10% (7–13) | 8% (5–11) |

Adapted with permission from the American Urological Association 2003.

TUMT, transurethral microwave thermotherapy; TUNA, transurethral needle ablation; TURP, transurethral resection of the prostate; UTI, urinary tract infection.

TABLE 6.6

## Outcomes of surgical therapies: estimates of median percentage rates of adverse events (95% confidence interval)

| | Acute urinary retention | BNC/ stricture | Hematuria, significant | Incontinence | Infection/ UTI | Secondary procedure | Sexual: ejaculation | Sexual: erectile problems | Transfusion |
|---|---|---|---|---|---|---|---|---|---|
| TURP | 5% (4–8) | 7% (5–8) | 6% (5–8) | 3% (2–5) | 6% (5–9) | 5% (4–6) | 65% (56–72) | 10% (7–13) | 8% (5–11) |
| HoLRP | 8% (2–17) | 5% (1–19) | 3% (1–9) | 1% (0–11) | 1% (0–11) | 1% (1–11) | 59% (37–79) | 3% (0–12) | 2% (0–7) |
| Transurethral laser coagulation | 21% (16–28) | 5% (3–7) | 3% (1–6) | 1% (0–3) | 9% (6–13) | 7% (5–9) | 17% (12–24) | 6% (3–12) | 2% (1–4) |
| TUIP | 6% (3–10) | 6% (4–10) | 5% (1–15) | 2% (1–6) | 5% (3–8) | 14% (8–22) | 18% (12–25) | 13% (6–23) | 3% (1–7) |
| Transurethral electrovaporization | 12% (7–17) | 5% (4–8) | 6% (3–9) | 3% (2–6) | 8% (4–15) | 8% (5–11) | 65% (43–83) | 8% (4–12) | 1% (1–3) |
| Transurethral laser vaporization | 13% (8–19) | 3% (1–6) | 10% (4–20) | 3% (1–6) | 9% (6–12) | 8% (5–11) | 42% (21–66) | 7% (4–11) | 3% (1–5) |
| Open prostatectomy | 1% (0–8) | 8% (2–17) | 1% (0–8) | 6% (1–20) | 8% (3–17) | 1% (0–8) | 61% (35–84) | – | 27% (23–32) |
| Active surveillance | 3% (2–6) | – | – | 2% (1–3) | 0% (0–1) | 55% (49–61) | – | 21% (17–26) | 0% (0–1) |

Adapted with permission from the American Urological Association 2003.

BNC, bladder neck contracture; HoLRP, holmium laser resection of the prostate; TUIP, transurethral incision of the prostate; TURP, transurethral resection of the prostate.

TABLE 6.7

**Changes in everyday activities due to BPH symptoms**

- Drinking before travel limited
- Drinking before bedtime restricted
- Driving for 2 hours without a break impossible
- Sleep disrupted
- Visiting places without toilets restricted
- Outdoor sports, such as golf, limited
- Many social activities, such as going to the cinema or theater, avoided

## Sexual function and BPH

Many men suffering from moderate to severe LUTS as a result of BPH are also troubled by associated sexual dysfunction. Therapy to improve BPH symptoms, especially with $\alpha_1$-blockers, seems to improve overall sexual function, although the mechanism for this is unclear. As the sympathetic nervous system is involved in the control of blood flow into the corpora cavernosa, it may be that part of this effect is achieved by the induction of smooth muscle relaxation within the erectile bodies (relaxation of the bladder neck, however, may cause retrograde ejaculation, a side effect seen particularly in those treated with tamsulosin). A recent study has also found that improvement in sexual function was more marked in a TURP group than in laser-treated patients. One possible explanation is that BPH sufferers may have such severe LUTS, including nocturia, that they feel disinclined to engage in sexual activity. As symptoms improve with either medical or surgical therapy the desire for intercourse may increase.

When a man is evaluated for BPH, inquiries about sexual dysfunction are certainly in order, especially since effective treatment with type-5 phosphodiesterase inhibitors (sildenafil, vardenafil or tadalafil) is now available. 5$\alpha$-reductase inhibitors (finasteride or dutasteride) carry a reversible 3–5% risk of reducing libido and erections, and should be used only after the patient has received an explanation of these side effects.

TABLE 6.8

**Reasons for unwillingness to seek medical help**

- Modification of lifestyle makes symptoms bearable
- Belief that symptoms are age-associated and need not be treated
- Fear of a diagnosis of cancer
- Unwillingness to undergo surgery, concern about complications
- Embarrassment about discussing symptoms, particularly with a female doctor
- Dislike of digital rectal examination
- Reluctance to go into hospital for treatment

---

**Key points – considerations in treatment decisions**

- BPH therapy should be selected using the 'balance-sheet' concept of efficacy versus side effects.
- Patient preference is an important consideration. Men with mild symptoms tend to opt for active surveillance; those with moderate or severe symptoms choose either medical or surgical therapy.
- The impact of any BPH therapy on sexual function is an important consideration.

---

**Key references**

American Urological Association. AUA guideline on management of benign prostatic hyperplasia (2003). *J Urol* 2003;170:530–47.

Brookes ST, Donovan JL, Peters TJ et al. Sexual dysfunction in men after treatment for lower urinary symptoms: evidence from randomised controlled trial. *BMJ* 2002;324: 1059–61.

Johnson NJ, Kirby RS. Treatments for benign prostatic hyperplasia: an analysis of their clinical and economic impact in the UK and Italy. *J Outcomes Res* 1999;3:11–26.

McConnell JD, Bruskewitz R, Walsh PC et al. The effect of finasteride on the risk of acute urinary retention and the need for surgical treatment among men with benign prostatic hyperplasia. Finasteride Long-Term Efficacy and Safety Study Group. *N Engl J Med* 1998;338:557–63.

Roehrborn C, Boyle P, Nickel J et al. ARIA3001 ARIA3002 and ARIA3003 Study Investigators. Efficacy and safety of a dual inhibitor of 5-alpha-reductase types 1 and 2 (dutasteride) in men with benign prostatic hyperplasia. *Urology* 2002;60:434–41.

Rosen R, Altwein J, Boyle P et al. Lower urinary tract symptoms and male sexual dysfunction: the multinational survey of the aging male (MSAM-7). *Eur Urol* 2003; 44:637–49.

The ancient Greek philosopher Heraclitus observed that the only constant is change. Currently, the management of BPH is undergoing radical change. In many disease areas, the shift continues from hospital-based surgical treatments towards medical therapies administered by primary care physicians. Such moves are of course encouraged by governments and insurers, who hold the purse-strings and perceive this trend as cost-efficient. While some urologists may regret the passing of the era when treatment decisions about BPH simply involved a choice between prostatectomy and active surveillance, new opportunities now exist for those who are prepared to grasp the future. Those who prefer the past are likely to find the world leaving them behind.

## Health economics

The cost–benefit implications of any emerging treatment that seems destined to be widely used are complex. Do medical therapies such as the anti-ulcer drugs save money by reducing the surgical intervention rate? More likely, they lead to escalation of costs as large numbers of individuals are treated who would probably never have come to surgery.

Counterbalancing this cost issue, however, is the health gain derived from the new treatment modality. Take the example of extracorporeal shockwave lithotripsy for renal stones; the machines may cost in excess of one million dollars and multiple treatments are sometimes needed, but the requirement for an open operation and hospitalization are avoided. Ask the average patient about their treatment preference and they will almost always opt for the non-invasive therapy, provided it is safe and effective; but the burden of cost for the treatment advance has, of course, to be borne either by the individual or society.

## A cascade of therapies?

Another concern for the future is the risk that many millions of men with BPH, instead of undergoing one-off definitive surgery, will be treated instead with a 'cascade' of less effective therapies: for example, first $\alpha_1$-blockers and/or finasteride, then thermotherapy, followed by laser therapy, before finally resorting to a standard TURP. Although such worries seem legitimate, patients themselves often prefer a stepwise approach.

More information is needed about the long-term efficacy and overall failure rate of the new competing therapies for BPH. It must be remembered that even TURP has a 16–20% incidence of need for further therapy over 8 years. Less invasive treatments seem likely to fail more often, although it has been pointed out that there are health-economic arguments in favor of deferring surgery, especially in a slowly progressive benign condition such as BPH. Pharmacotherapy for BPH is also improving in both safety and efficacy, and has now been conclusively shown to improve quality of life and delay disease progression, especially when used in combination, as in the MTOPS study.

## Concerns for undiagnosed prostate cancer

One of the advantages of TURP is the yield of resected tissue that can be evaluated histologically to identify prostate cancer (present in around 10% of TURP). Neither medical nor minimally invasive treatment options permit this. In fact, about two-thirds of these so-called incidental cancers are T1a low-volume tumors that have little or no impact on overall survival and usually do not require therapy. Identification of these tumors by TURP may therefore only serve to alarm both the patient and the clinician unnecessarily. The remaining one-third (affecting just 3% of men undergoing TURP) are higher volume, less well-differentiated T1b tumors, for which therapy may be indicated in younger men. Fortunately, most of these cancers can be pre-identified by DRE and PSA testing, and the diagnosis confirmed by ultrasound-guided prostatic biopsy, so that the risks of missing significant, life-threatening cancers are probably small overall.

Indeed, the increased surveillance of more patients treated medically seems likely to result in an increase rather than a decrease in the diagnosis of localized prostate cancer. It should, however, be noted that TURP should never be carried out merely to exclude a diagnosis of prostate cancer.

## Shared care: the way forward

The increasing involvement of primary care physicians in the diagnosis and management of BPH is a constructive initiative that should be viewed positively, because in fact several advantages may arise from it. Urologists will be free to devote more time to patients with more complex and life-threatening conditions, such as prostate cancer. Family physicians will be able to care more comprehensively for men beyond middle age, and patients will be spared the inconvenience of repeated hospital visits for this progressive and bothersome but seldom life-threatening condition.

However, before primary care physicians can assume this role, there are a number of procedures to master and treatment options to appreciate (Table 7.1), all of which have been described in the preceding pages. This can only be accomplished by closer interaction between urologists and their local primary care physicians – a process termed 'shared care'. Urologists of the 21st century must be prepared to inform and educate their colleagues about prostatic disease and how shared care can work. They must also make themselves aware of holistic issues in men's health and treat the patient as a whole, not just the prostate as an independent entity.

TABLE 7.1

**The primary care physician's knowledge checklist for managing BPH**

- Case finding
- Prostate-specific antigen
- Flow rate
- Treatment options
- International Prostate Symptom Score
- Digital rectal examination technique
- Post-void residual urine
- Follow-up

Closer interaction with local urologists will expedite the learning process as well as help to establish new and better protocols

As the information technology revolution affects all of us more and more, doctor–patient interactions will be increasingly 'virtual', based on the computer, internet and telemedicine links.

The days of patients with BPH needing to travel frequently to large and impersonal hospital clinics are rapidly drawing to a close. The challenge for urologists and primary care physicians, now and in the future, is to work together to reduce the quality-of-life impairment and suffering associated with this most prevalent disease of elderly men. There is also important work to do to raise awareness of men's health issues in general and the problem of BPH in particular. The authors hope that the fifth edition of this book will support the process.

# Useful addresses

American Urological Association
1000 Corporate Blvd
Linthicum, Maryland 21090
USA
Tel: 866 746 4282 (toll free)
Tel: 410 689 3700
Fax: 410 689 3800
www.auanet.org
www.auanet.org/guidelines/
bph.cfm (BPH guidelines)

American Foundation for Urologic
Disease
1000 Corporate Blvd, Suite 410
Linthicum, Maryland 21090
USA
Tel: 800 828 7866 (toll free)
www.afud.org

National Kidney and Urologic
Diseases Information
Clearinghouse
3 Information Way
Bethesda, MD 20892-3580
USA
Tel: 800 891 5390 or
301 654 4415
Fax: 301 907 8906
nkudic@info.niddk.nih.gov
kidney.niddk.nih.gov

American Academy of Family
Physicians BPH website
familydoctor.org/x2282.xml

Urotoday website
www.urotoday.com

British Urological Foundation
35–43 Lincoln's Inn Fields
London WC2 3PE UK
info@buf.org.uk
www.buf.org.uk

European Association of Urology
PO Box 30016
6803 AA Arnhem
The Netherlands
Tel: +31 (0)26 389 06 80
Fax: +31 (0)26 389 06 74
eau@uroweb.nl
www.uroweb.com

Prostate Research Campaign UK
10 Northfields Prospect
Putney Bridge Road
London SW18 1PE UK
Tel: 020 8877 5840
info@prostate-research.org.uk
www.prostate-research.org.uk

Sexual Dysfunction Association
Windmill Place Business Centre
2-4 Windmill Lane, Southall
Middlesex UB2 4NJ UK
Tel: 0870 7743571
info@sda.uk.net
www.sda.uk.net

The Continence Foundation
307 Hatton Square
16 Baldwins Gardens
London ECIN 7RJ UK
Helpline 0845 345 0165
(Mon–Fri 9:30–13:00)
continence-help@dial.pipex.com
www.continence-foundation.
org.uk

# Index

treatment decisions 8,
32–3, 73–81, 83, 85
cost-effectiveness 73
likelihood of
complications 73, 74,
75–6, 77–9, 81
long-term efficacy 73, 74,
75, 84
patient preference 73,
74–6, 81
risk of progression 73, 74
severity of symptoms 73
triglycerides 42
tuberculosis 16
type-5 phosphodiesterase
inhibitors 80

ultrasound-guided prostatic
biopsy 84
see also transabdominal
ultrasound; transrectal
ultrasound

unwillingness to consult
doctor 76, 81
urethral stricture 22
urethrocystoscopy 34
urge incontinence 5, 22
urgency 5, 14, 16, 22, 23,
60
urinalysis 21, 25–6, 33, 34,
53
urinary retention 5, 65, 69
see also acute; chronic
urinary tract infection
(UTI) 16, 25, 50, 57, 60,
67, 78, 79
urine cytology see
urinalysis
urine microscopy see
urinalysis
urodynamics 31–2, 33, 34,
44
uroflowmetry 29, 30, 33,
34

uroselectivity 43

vardenafil 80
Veteran's Administration
Cooperative Study 49, 50
visual laser ablation of the
prostate (VLAP) 6
see also ELAP

watchful waiting see active
surveillance
weak flow/stream 5, 14,
21, 22, 23, 33

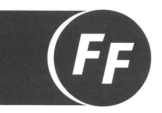

# FAST FACTS

## An outstandingly successful independent medical handbook series

### *Over one million copies sold*

- Written by world experts
- Concise and practical
- Up-to-date
- Designed for ease of reading and reference
- Copiously illustrated with useful photographs, diagrams and charts

Our aim for *Fast Facts* remains the same as ever: to be **the world's most respected medical handbook series**. Feedback on how to make titles even more useful is always welcome (feedback@fastfacts.com).

## *Fast Facts* titles include

Acne
Allergic Rhinitis
Asthma (second edition)
Benign Gynecological Disease (second edition)
Bipolar Disorder
Brain Tumors
Breast Cancer (second edition)
Celiac Disease
Chronic Obstructive Pulmonary Disease
Colorectal Cancer (second edition)
Contraception
Dementia
Depression
Disorders of the Hair and Scalp
Dyspepsia (second edition)
Eczema and Contact Dermatitis
Endometriosis (second edition)
Epilepsy (second edition)
Erectile Dysfunction (third edition)
Gynecological Oncology
Headaches (second edition)

Hyperlipidemia (second edition)
Hypertension (second edition)
Inflammatory Bowel Disease
Irritable Bowel Syndrome (second edition)
Menopause
Minor Surgery
Multiple Sclerosis
Osteoporosis (fourth edition)
Parkinson's Disease
Prostate Specific Antigen (second edition)
Psoriasis
Respiratory Tract Infection (second edition)
Rheumatoid Arthritis
Schizophrenia (second edition)
Sexual Dysfunction
Sexually Transmitted Infections
Soft Tissue Rheumatology
Superficial Fungal Infections
Travel Medicine
Urinary Continence (second edition)
Urinary Stones

## Orders

To order via the website, or to find regional distributors, please go to
www.fastfacts.com

For telephone orders, please call +44 (0)1752 202301 (UK) or
800 538 1287 (North America, toll free)